Analytical Case Studies on Municipal and Biomedical Waste Management

Effective waste management practices are essential to mitigate unfavourable impacts and achieve the Sustainable Development Goals. This book covers perspectives addressing the Sustainable Development Goals through analytical and case studies on municipal and biomedical waste management. It consists of ten selectively curated highly technical chapters covering various aspects of achieving the Sustainable Development Goals through applying effective waste management strategies and practices through practical case studies and examples.

Features:

- Analysis of over 30 real-life case studies reviewed from local as well as global perspectives.
- Discusses application of technologies in real time.
- Addresses the 17 Sustainable Development Goals at ground level.
- Covers a broad range of case studies on municipal solid waste and biomedical waste treatment and management.
- Reviews the latest evidence-based approach in diagnosis and management.

This book is aimed at researchers and graduate students in environmental engineering and management.

Analytical Case Studies on Municipal and Biomedical Waste Management

Perspectives on Sustainable Development Goals

Edited by Moharana Choudhury, Ankur Rajpal, Srijan Goswami, Arghya Chakravorty and Vimala Raghavan

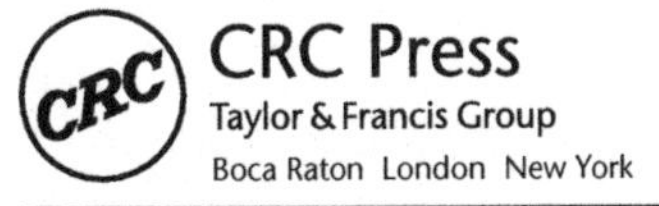

CRC Press
Taylor & Francis Group
Boca Raton London New York

CRC Press is an imprint of the Taylor & Francis Group, an **informa** business

First edition published 2025
by CRC Press
2385 NW Executive Center Drive, Suite 320, Boca Raton FL 33431

and by CRC Press
4 Park Square, Milton Park, Abingdon, Oxon, OX14 4RN

CRC Press is an imprint of Taylor & Francis Group, LLC

ISBN: 978-1-032-79691-8 (hbk)
ISBN: 978-1-032-81406-3 (pbk)
ISBN: 978-1-003-49969-5 (ebk)

DOI: 10.1201/9781003499695

Typeset in Times
by Apex CoVantage, LLC

Contents

Foreword

I am delighted to read the book *Analytical Case Studies on Municipal and Biomedical Waste Management*. Waste management has become a necessity for human beings, especially in the municipality area and biomedical field. Inadequate waste management practices are not just threats to the environment at large but also catalyse the spread of infectious diseases through secondary transmission. Thus, to win the battle against this disruptive problem, adopting efficient and harmless waste disposal strategies is necessary.

The book focuses on the issue of the waste management sector during the epidemic and discusses various case studies of municipal and biomedical waste management in different countries for sustainable development. Also, the book specializes in applications of COVID-19–associated biomedical waste management issues and solutions for the global research community. The editorial team has given their best effort and concisely emphasized the basic and advanced concepts. The concept of the book is straightforward, and the technical depth is kept balanced to be understood by the young scientific community as well as established researchers in this field.

The book is a mine of information, demonstrating the techniques in minutest detail; it is a source of inspiration and information for those who work in the same domain. The technical depth and knowledge covered by the book delighted me, and I could not simply stop myself from attending it. In short, this book is unique and surely a work to treasure for anyone who works in the field of waste management. So read it, enjoy it, and learn from it. I feel like this will be a tonic stimulant for the flow of knowledge in its field. This book will not only become beneficial for academicians or researchers but also will help to enhance the proficiency of waste management employees. I would like to compliment the editors, authors, and co-authors for producing such a masterpiece.

I hope that this book will inspire and empower readers to embark on a journey of discovery, innovation, and collective action, as we strive to address one of the defining challenges of our time: the responsible stewardship of our planet's finite resources.

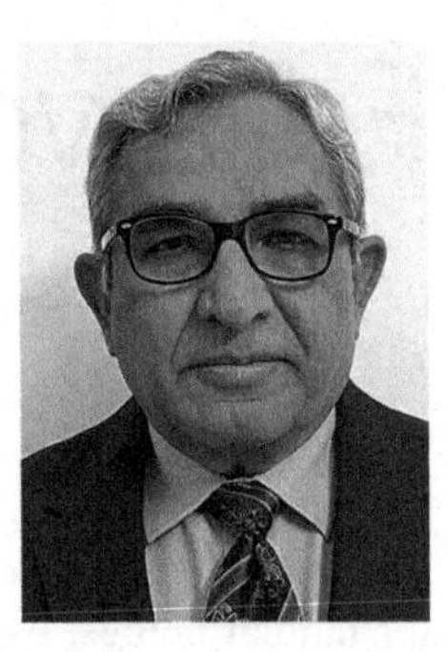

Professor Ashok Pandey
PhD, FBRS, FTWAS, FNASc, FNA, FRSB,
FIOBB, FAMI, FISEES, FICS, FWSSET
BRSI Distinguished Fellow
HTBS National Innovation Chair
UPES Distinguished Professor
KHU Korea Eminent Scholar
IIT Roorkee Visiting Professor

Distinguished Scientist
Centre for Innovation and Translational Research
CSIR-Indian Institute of Toxicology Research
Lucknow-226 001, India

Preface

In the present state of the environment, the exponential rise in industrialization and urbanization has resulted in the contamination of the air one breathes, the water one drinks, and even the food and the soil and water in which the food grows. Environmental contamination has also resulted from various industrial operations like fugitive emissions, accidental spills, leaks, and dumping of hazardous substances. These are the consequences of using synthetic organic chemicals such as solvents, pesticides, refrigerants, and chemical intermediates. Over the years, the excessive use of these synthetic chemicals, which are not degradable by natural means, has become hazardous or toxic. Unlike industrial and household wastes, biomedical wastes (BMW) are hazardous and serve as a potential source of pathogens. BMW are those wastes generated during the treatment of infected persons and usually comprise solid, liquid, or laboratory waste. Untreated medical waste harms both human health and the environment. Recently, the novel coronavirus had unprecedented implications for most of the world's countries. Also, in middle- and low-income countries, household medical waste due to ongoing home healthcare treatment and lack of COVID waste disposal awareness, such as masks, disposable vaccination syringes, and protective gear, is just dumped without following the prescribed guidelines. So far, preventive measures such as raising medical standards, aggressive testing campaigns, and regulating public policies have been implemented to combat this public health disaster. The proper identification, assortment, separation, storage, transportation, treatment, and disposal of biological and healthcare waste, as well as critical connected factors like proper sanitization, training, and protection of waste collection workforces, are all essential components of effective waste management practices. Inadequate waste management practices are not just threats to the environment at large but also catalyse the spread of SARS-CoV-2 or any other infectious diseases through secondary transmission. Thus, to win the battle against the upcoming pandemic, adopting efficient and harmless waste disposal strategies is necessary. Countries across the globe have adopted individual stringent measures to tackle contamination levels and subsequent waste management; however, these measures need to be revised. In addition to this, the World Health Organization (WHO) has recently set out COVID-19 waste management guidelines, but their implementation depends upon the country's context.

On the other hand, global solid waste generation is increasing enormously, and the annual waste generation rate is anticipated to rise by 70% from 2.01 billion tonnes in 2016 to around 3.40 billion tonnes in 2050. With the continued increase in waste generation, the problem of waste management grows threefold, and disposal in landfills is thus the most economical way to eliminate it. However, landfills are the third largest and fastest-growing source of methane emissions globally. An accurate prediction of landfill gas (LFG) emission and recovery will advance the knowledge used to select an appropriate municipal solid waste (MSW) treatment technology and LFG emission reduction strategies in the future. Hence, vital case studies are presented here to elaborate on the accurate prediction of LFG emission and knowledge for appropriate municipal solid waste treatment technology and LFG emission reduction strategies in the future. This edited volume provides comprehensive, insightful information. It focuses on the waste management sector's issues during the epidemic and discusses various case studies of municipal and biomedical waste management in different countries focused on Sustainable Development Goals (SDGs). Also, the book specializes in applications of COVID-19–associated biomedical waste management issues and solutions for the readers. The editorial team has given their best effort and concisely emphasized basic and advanced concepts. This edited collection represents the combined efforts of the editorial team, all the contributing authors, and the peer reviewer panel from reputed institutions and organizations worldwide.

The Editors

About the Editors

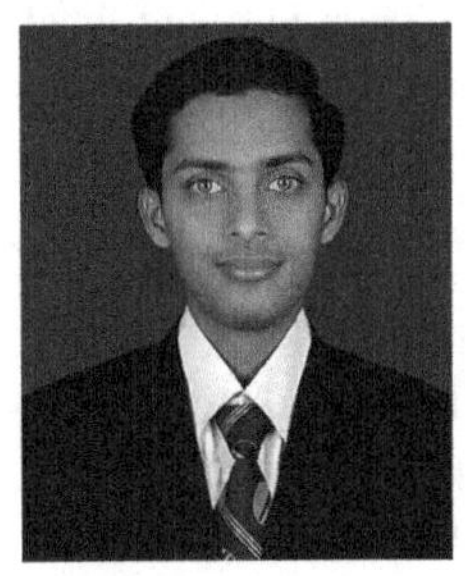

Moharana Choudhury is a researcher and environmentalist from Guwahati, Assam, India. He has completed his education as an MSc, PGDGIS, PGDEM, and PGCGARD from Gurukul Kangri Deemed to be University, Haridwar, Uttarakhand, India; North Eastern Hill University (NEHU), Shillong Meghalaya, India; and Tezpur University, Assam and National Institute of Rural Development (NIRD) Hyderabad, India, respectively. Choudhury has worked on various scientific projects in various government departments and has more than 12 years of research and working experience in the field of the environment. He began his career as a research intern at the National Institute of Disaster Management (NIDM) in New Delhi, followed by the North Eastern Space Application Center (Department of Space, Government of India/ISRO Unit) as a junior research fellow. Choudhury has authored or edited five books with internationally reputed publications, more than 33 articles in national and internationally reputed journals and proceedings, and more than 26 book chapters. He has written many articles and scientific reports in popular magazines. Choudhury is working on various environmental conservation activities in Assam and the country. He has worked on several initiatives to integrate environmentally sustainable projects for iconic heritage places, wetlands, and ecotourism spots in Assam, India, especially for cleanliness waste management and beating single-use plastic pollution-related projects. He contributes to various environmental research, management, social media mass awareness, and research studies. He is also well known in India for his efforts to implement environmental education and safeguard the privileges of environmental degree holders in India.

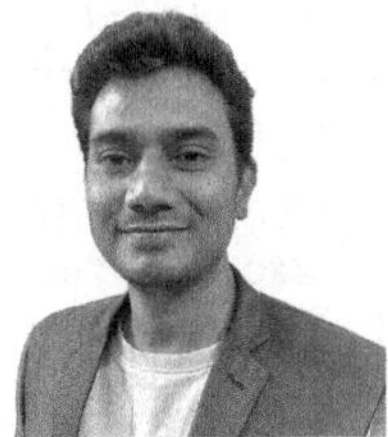

Ankur Rajpal holds a PhD in environmental science (2011), and currently he is working as Project Scientist-C and responsible for international and national wastewater, sludge and solid waste management-related projects in the Indian Institute of Technology Roorkee (IITR), India. Earlier, he worked at the Honk Kong Baptist University (HKBU) Hong Kong as a postdoc fellow. He also worked as Senior Research Fellow in the Central Pollution Control Board (CPCB), MoEF, Delhi, India. Dr. Rajpal is a fellow and life member of several professional bodies and organizations such as IWA and ANSF. In the past years, he has published more than 30 peer-reviewed articles in international journals. He is an active reviewer of several international journals and has participated in more than 25 international and national conferences. His research achievements include many academic honours. He received two best poster awards, and recently, he received the Young Scientist award, 2019, from national-level agencies. His research interest is focused on problems related to wastewater and bio-waste treatment, enhancement of nutrient recovery, and micro-pollutant removal from waste and wastewater.

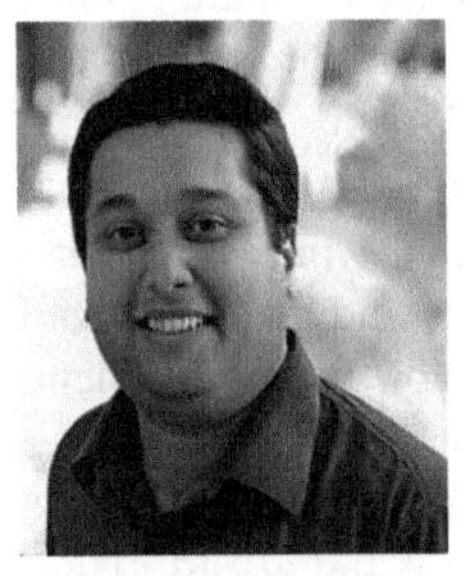

Srijan Goswami is Author and Editor of several medical science books (PG-Research category), as well as Research Scholar at Department of Biotechnology, University of North Bengal, India, and Research Coordinator at Biomedical and Allied Sciences Division, Voice of Environment, Assam, India. He is a physician of the biochemic system of medicine and also holds specialization in medical biotechnology and clinical nutrition. He received his professional training on community nutrition and child care, medical microbiology, medical biochemistry, and diabetes counselling from reputed medical colleges in Kolkata, India. He is experienced in teaching at diverse range of paramedical and life sciences departments of reputed colleges and institutions. He is presently Research Coordinator, Biomedical Research and Allied Sciences Division, Voice of Environment, Assam, India. Dr. Goswami has around 11 years of experience in the field of teaching and research and has published four books (with ten in the pipeline) and ~40 research papers in national and international journals. He has independently and successfully guided around ten undergraduate and postgraduate students to complete their research work and publications in the past three years. Dr. Goswami has received four Letters of Commendation for Global Community Services and Certificate of Honor for his contribution in the field of science and knowledge from the *International Journal of Agricultural Research, Sustainability and Food Sufficiency* (IJARSFS), *International Journal of Advances in Medical Sciences and Biotechnology* (IJAMSB), and *International Journal of Health, Safety and Environment* (IJHSE) in 2019, 2020, 2021, and 2023. The *Current Research in Nutrition and Food Science* (Enviro Research Group) and *Academia Scholarly Journals* awarded him the Certificate of Excellence as a reviewer in 2020, 2021, and 2023. He is actively associated with the editorial review boards of 15 international journals.

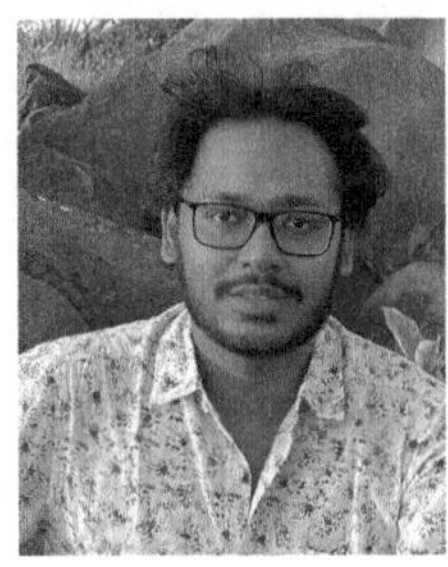

Arghya Chakravorty is an early career, young, passionate researcher and enthusiastic active member of the American Chemical Society, Solid Waste Association of North America, and British Society for Antimicrobial Chemotherapy, as well as a registered doctoral fellow at the Centre for Nanotechnology Research, Vellore Institute of Technology—Vellore, India, holding four Indian patents, while his research interest is interdisciplinary material science and nanobiotechnology. He also likes to deal with different aspects of human resources and professional relationships. He has contributed to editing five books for Springer Nature, CRC Press, and Taylor & Francis; a dozen book chapters for different renowned international publishers like Elsevier, Springer, CRC Press, and IGI Global–USA; and a couple of research as well as review papers. He has been added as a reviewer of several international standard books and reputed peer-reviewed SCI journals and awarded several national and international recognitions.

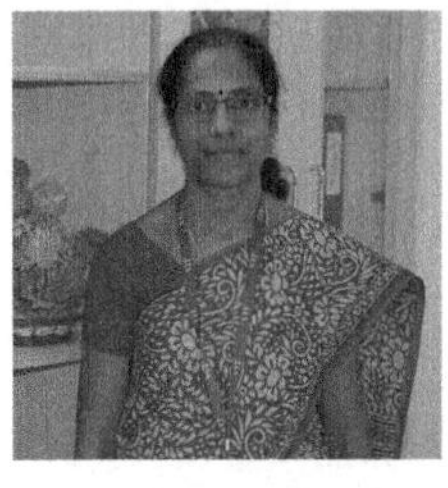

Vimala Raghavan is an enthusiastic and innovative associate professor at the Centre for Nanotechnology Research, Vellore Institute of Technology (VIT), Vellore, India, and has an h-index (Google Scholar) of 19. She received her PhD in environmental biotechnology from VIT, Vellore, India. She has guest-edited several special issues of SCI- and SCOPUS-indexed journals, while her research interest is in various niche areas of nanotechnology like hybrid nanobiomaterials; synthesis; and applications in therapeutics, diagnostics, environmental remediation, and the energy sector. She has guided three PhD scholars, and ten master's project students. She is currently guiding six PhD scholars, as well as serving as an investigator of several internationally and nationally funded research projects. She has more than 50 international and national journal publications and has contributed three book chapters and many conference papers.

Contributors

Daisy Alexander
Manipal Law School
Manipal Academy of Higher Education
Bengaluru Campus
India

Nithiya Anbuselvam
IBDP Biology and IP Biology Teacher
Department of Science
Hwa Chong International School
Singapore

Tsering Angmo
Indian Institute of Integrative Medicine
Canal Road, Jammu-180001
India

Sudipti Arora
Dr. B. Lal Institute of Biotechnology
Malviya Industrial Area
Malviya Nagar, Jaipur
India

Rajdeep Banerjee
Rajendra Memorial Research Institute of Medical Sciences
Patna-800007
India
Centre for Cancer Research
National Cancer Institute, Bethesda, MD
USA

Sunanda Chandaa
Agricultural and Ecological Research Unit
Indian Statistical Institute Kolkata-700108
India

Pradeep Das
National Institute of Cholera and Enteric Diseases
Kolkata-700010
India

Sukhendu Dey
Department of Environmental Science
The University of Burdwan
West Bengal
India

Saurabh Dhakad
Jawaharlal Nehru University
New Delhi
India

Kanwarpal S Dhugga
International Maize and Wheat Improvement Center (CIMMYT)
Texcoco 56237
Mexico

Pallavi Gahlot
Environmental Biotechnology Group
Department of Civil Engineering
Indian Institute of Technology Roorkee
Roorkee-247667
India

Sandipan Ganguly
National Institute of Cholera and Enteric Diseases
Kolkata-700010
India

Apurba Ratan Ghosh
Department of Environmental Science
The University of Burdwan
West Bengal
India

Nilofer Hussaini
School of Commerce, Finance and Accounting
Christ University
Bangalore
India

Tajwar Hussaini
Amity University
Academic City
Dubai
UAE

Sunitha Abhay Jain
School of Law
Christ University
India

Sunil John
Manipal Law School
Manipal Academy of Higher Education
Bengaluru Campus
India

Ajay Jose
Molecular Medicine and Pathology
University of Auckland
Auckland-1023
New Zealand

Phinu Mary Jose
School of Business and Management
Central Campus
Bangalore
India

Seena Thomas K
Department of Statistics
Christ University
Central Campus
Bangalore
India

Sunaja Devi K R
Department of Chemistry
Christ (Deemed to be University)
Bangalore-560029
Karnataka
India

Mani Lakshmi
Centre for Environmental Studies
Lady Doak College
Madurai, Tamil Nadu
India

Parameswaran Kiruthika Lakshmi
Department of Microbiology
The Madura College
Madurai, Tamil Nadu
India

Nishu Mittal
Institute of Biosciences and Technology
Shri Ram Swaroop Memorial University
Lucknow-225003
India

Md. Moniruzzaman
Institute of Nuclear Science & Technology
Bangladesh Atomic Energy Commission
Dhaka
Bangladesh

Shabarisha N
School of Business and Management
Christ University
Bannerghatta Road Campus
Pai Layout, Hulimavu
Bangalore
India

Sarangapani Nivarthi
Associate Professor
CMS, Business School
JAIN (Deemed to be University)
Bangalore
India

Dephan Pinheiro
Department of Chemistry
Christ (Deemed to be University)
Bangalore-560029
Karnataka
India

Gowri Shankar R
School of Business and Management
Christ University
Bannerghatta Road Campus
Pai Layout, Hulimavu
Bangalore
India

Madhushree R
Department of Chemistry
Christ (Deemed to be University)
Bangalore-560029
Karnataka
India

Abdul Rafey
Department of Chemical Engineering
Aligarh Muslim University
Aligarh
India

Vasudevan Rajaram
Oak Brook, Illinois
USA

Shweta Rajpal
Era's Lucknow Medical College & Hospital
Lucknow, Uttar Pradesh 226003
India

Pandi Sakthieaswari
Department of Botany & Microbiology
Lady Doak College
Madurai, Tamil Nadu
India

Vikas Janardhan Salunkhe
CMS Business School
JAIN University
Bangalore
India

Palas Samanta
Department of Environmental Science
Sukanta Mahavidyalaya
University of North Bengal
West Bengal
India

Bidisha Sarkar
School of Business & Management
Christ University
Bangalore
India

Sutripta Sarkar
Agricultural and Ecological Research Unit
Indian Statistical Institute
Kolkata-700108
India
Barrackpore Rastraguru Surendranath College
Kolkata-700120
India

Sonika Saxena
University of Adelaide
Adelaide SA 5005
Australia

Faisal Zia Siddiqui
Department of Chemical Engineering
Aligarh Muslim University
Aligarh
India

Tauseef Zia Siddiqui
Sustainability & Environmental Analyst
Qatargas
Qatar

Darshan SM
Department of Mechanical and Automobile Engineering
Christ University
Bangalore
India

Devanshi Sutaria
University of Adelaide
Australia

Chockaiyan Usha
Department of Zoology & Microbiology
Thiagarajar College
Madurai, Tamil Nadu
India

Global Energy Potential of Landfill Gas

1

Abdul Rafey, Faisal Zia Siddiqui, and Tauseef Zia Siddiqui

1.1 INTRODUCTION

According to UNEP 2021, fossil fuels, waste, and agriculture are the three sectors that generate the most anthropogenic methane (CH_4). Oil and gas contribute 23% of emissions in the fossil fuel sector, while coal mining accounts for 12%. In the waste sector, landfills and wastewater account for 20% of emissions (UNEP, 2021). The World Bank estimates that in 2016, around 2,000 million tonnes of municipal solid waste (MSW) were generated, and this is projected to rise to about 3,400 million tonnes by 2050 (Kaza et al., 2018), which is likely to be a major challenge for governments and policymakers across the world. Landfill disposal is considered a primary waste disposal method among the various waste disposal methods in most countries, whether developed or developing economies (Mondal et al., 2023; Kaza et al., 2018). Around 70% of all MSW generated is globally disposed of in secured and unsecured landfills (Fischedick et al., 2014; Kaza et al., 2018). Waste disposal in landfills is the primary technique to dispose of MSW globally; more than 740 million tonnes of MSW are disposed of annually in landfills, amounting to 37% of the total global MSW generation. The USA and China are the top waste generators, with around 3,000 operational landfills (Rueda-Avellaneda et al., 2021). According to USEPA 2021, landfills disposing of MSW are the

DOI: 10.1201/9781003499695-1

third largest source of methane (CH_4) emissions in the USA, emitting approximately 99.4 million tonnes of carbon dioxide (CO_2) equivalent (MMTCO_2e) in the atmosphere in the year 2019. Methane is a significant emission from landfills that can be recovered as an energy source, leading to an offset in fossil fuel-based energy production(Manfredi et al., 2009). In the US, 435 landfills recovered around 7.1 billion m^3 LFG, and the electricity generation by these plants was around 10.5 billion kWh, equivalent to powering 8,10,000 homes and heating 547 billion (Guzzone & Leatherwood, 2007). Based on these facts, research and development efforts towards landfill gas (LFG) to energy recovery have taken a fast track.

1.1.1 Selected Global LFG to Electricity Generation Projects

Cited in Table 1.1 are 8 case studies of successful/operational LFG to electricity generation projects worldwide.

It is evident from the selected LFG to electricity generation projects that the amount of energy generation, as well as the reduction in the emissions, is directly dependent on the type of project chosen: gas turbine, cogeneration, reciprocating engine, steam turbine, microturbine, or combined cycle.

1.1.2 Selected Global LFG to Direct Use Projects

Cited in Table 1.2 are 8 case studies of successful/operational LFG to direct energy use projects worldwide.

It is evident from the LFG to direct use projects that the amount of energy generation, as well as the reduction in emissions, are directly dependent on the type of project chosen: direct thermal application, boilers, leachate evaporation, or greenhouse activities.

1.1.3 Selected Global LFG to Flaring Projects

Cited in Table 1.3 are five case studies of successful/operational LFG to flaring projects worldwide.

It is evident from the LFG to flaring projects that the amount of gas flow rate and the reduction in the emissions are directly dependent on the capacity of the flare station/blower as well as the number of extraction wells used on the landfill site for gas collection.

TABLE 1.1 Selected LFG to Electricity Generation Projects Worldwide

LANDFILL NAME	*COUNTY*	*LANDFILL OPENING YEAR*	*LANDFILL CLOSING YEAR*	*WASTE IN PLACE (TONNES)*	*WASTE IN PLACE YEAR*	*LFG COLLECTED (MMSCFD)*	*PROJECT START YEAR*	*TYPE OF LFG TO ENERGY PROJECT*	*ENERGY GENERATION (MW)*	*LFG FLOW TO PROJECT (MMSCFD)*	*EMISSION REDUCTION (MMTCO2E/YR)—DIRECT*
Central LF	Providence	1955	2030	3,90,02,254	2019	13.93	2013	Combined cycle	32.8	—	1.4819
Arbor Hills Landfill Inc.	Washtenaw	1970	2028	6,64,55,203	2019	13.905	1996	Combined cycle	23.5	—	1.0617
Puente Hills LF	Los Angeles	1957	2013	14,22,50,454	2013	22.387	2016	Steam turbine	24	24.5	1.0843
Orange County SLF	Orange			3,29,54,638	2019	5.352	2011	Steam turbine	8	5.63	0.3614
Frank R. Bowerman SLF	Orange	1990	2053	5,76,81,443	2019	13.2	2016	Reciprocating engine	22.4	10.75	1.0120
Lorain County Landfill I & II	Lorain	1972	2036	4,13,59,122	2019	11.76	2011	Reciprocating engine	16	—	0.7229
Sunshine Canyon Landfill	Los Angeles	1955	2037	6,52,07,800	2019	26.158	2014	Gas turbine	20	10.24	0.9036
Livingston LF	Livingston	1978	2047	5,37,83,549	2019	10.559	2013	Gas turbine	15	8.5	0.6777

TABLE 1.2 Selected LFG to Direct Energy Use Projects Worldwide

LANDFILL NAME	*COUNTY*	*LANDFILL OPENING YEAR*	*LANDFILL CLOSING YEAR*	*WASTE IN PLACE (TONNES)*	*WASTE IN PLACE YEAR*	*LFG COLLECTED (MMSCFD)*	*PROJECT START YEAR*	*TYPE OF LFG TO ENERGY PROJECT*	*LFG FLOW TO PROJECT (MMSCFD)*	*CURRENT YEAR EMISSION REDUCTIONS (MMTCO2E/YR)—DIRECT*
Conestoga LF	Berks	1994	2052	3,51,87,511	2019	11.52	2008	Direct thermal	3.6	0.3152
Lanchester LF	Lancaster	1975	2029	1,49,12,007	2019	5.76	2004	Direct thermal	3.456	0.3026
Jefferson Parish SLF	Jefferson	1982	2050	1,53,03,544	2019	1.747	2009	Direct thermal	1.88	0.1646
McCarty Road LF	Harris	1972	2031	9,79,83,501	2019	13.821	2009	Boiler	2.99	0.2618
National Serv-All LF	Allen	1966	2058	2,10,08,766	2019	6.167	2002	Boiler	2.52	0.2206
South Side Landfill Inc.	Marion	1971	2039	2,39,57,886	2019	7.2	1999	Boiler	2.4	0.2101
Richland County Landfill	Richland	1972	2043	2,11,51,184	2019	4.053	2016	Leachate evaporation	0.92	0.0805
Oakridge Landfill Inc.	Dorchester	1987	2043	1,51,49,999	2019	2.043	2018	Leachate evaporation	0.86	0.0753

TABLE 1.3 Selected LFG to Flaring Projects Worldwide

LANDFILL NAME	*COUNTY*	*LANDFILL OPENING YEAR*	*LANDFILL CLOSING YEAR*	*WASTE IN PLACE (MG)*	*TOTAL WASTE FOOTPRINT (HA)*	*COLLECTION SYSTEM STARTUP*	*EXTRACTION WELLS*	*BLOWER/FLARE STATION CAPACITY (M^3/HR)*	*AVERAGE GAS FLOW IN 2010 (M^3/HR)*	*EMISSION REDUCTION IN 2010 (TONNES CO_2E)*
Buenos Aires	Argentina	2005	2010	15,000,000	82.5	March 2008	270	13,000	9,200 at 58% CH_4	669,600
Curva De Rodas	Colombia	1984	2003	8,500,000	33	July 2008	84	c3,000	634 at 37% CH_4	24,349
La Pradera	Colombia	2003	2027	3,500,000	30	December 2008	45	2,000	1465 at 50% CH_4	179,574
Guanajuato	Mexico	2001	2017	8,500,000	60	2009	48	1,869	310	178,901
Mariupol	Ukraine	1967	2008	2,100,000	12.3	February 2010	43	160–800	390 at 50% CH_4	40,000–75,000

1.2 PARAMETERS AFFECTING MSW DECOMPOSITION AND LFG EMISSION IN LANDFILLS

Table 1.4 summarizes various parameters affecting MSW decomposition and LFG emission in landfills. The table highlights the comprehensive research, indicating the main factors that increase and decrease LFG generation over the life span of MSW in a landfill.

1.2.1 Energy Potential of LFG per Unit of MSW

The energy of one m^3 LFG (50% CH_4) is approximately $0.5\,m^3$ of natural gas, 1.41 kg charcoal, 3.45 kg firewood, 0.79 litres petrol, 0.51 litres diesel/fuel/heating oil, 0.63 litres kerosene, or 4 to 5 KWh energy. LFG contains CH_4, which is combustible in nature. The combustion of CH_4 proceeds per the given reaction:

$$CH_4 + 2O_2 \rightarrow CO_2 + 2H_2O \; \Delta H = -890\,kJ/mole$$

1 m^3 methane on combustion at STP/NTP (25 dm^3) produces 1 m^3 of CH_4 = (890 / 0.025) kJ = 35,600 kJ of energy

One molar mass of biodegradable waste ($C_6H_{12}O_6$) = 180 g

One mole of CH_4 occupies 25 dm^3 at NTP

Then one mole of organic waste (180 g) produces 75 dm^3 of CH_4

One kg of waste generates $417\,dm^3$ of CH_4; therefore, 1 tonne of waste will produce $417\,m^3$ CH_4. Considering 30 – 40% of MSW is decomposable in nature, around 1 tonne of MSW will generate $170\,m^3$ of CH_4. The energy potential of LFG per unit of MSW assessed by various researchers is summarized year-wise in Table 1.5.

1.2.2 Energy Content of LFG and Methane

Table 1.6 summarizes the reported energy content of LFG and methane.

The higher calorific value can be obtained if the percentage of methane is higher in LFG. The application of LFG as an energy source depends on the extent of LFG extraction, treatment, and utilization. It can be categorized into three types based on the quality of LFG recovered, as shown in Table 1.7.

TABLE 1.4 Summary of Parameters Affecting MSW Decomposition and LFG Emission in Landfills

S.NO.	*PARAMETERS*	*INCREASE IN LFG GENERATION*	*DECREASE IN LFG GENERATION*	*REFERENCE*
1.	Large quantity of rapidly degradable MSW	Y		(Rettenberger & Stegmann, 1996)
2.	Higher organic content in MSW	Y		(Emcon Associates, 1980)
3.	Older age of MSW		Y	(El-Fadel & Rashed, 1998)
4.	Higher density of MSW	Y		(Nastev et al., 2001)
5.	Shredding/size reduction of MSW	Y		(Tittlebaum, 1982)
6.	Increased compaction of MSW	Y		(Buivid et al., 1981)
7.	Increased landfill depth	Y		(El-Fadel et al., 1996)
8.	Increased landfill temperature	Y 32–35 °C 34–38 °C 20–40 °C 41 °C 40 °C		(Gardner & Probert, 1993)
9.	Neutral pH of MSW	Y 6 to 8 6.4 to 7.2 7.0 to 7.2 6.4 to 7.4		(EHRIG, 1983)
10.	Increased moisture content of MSW	Y 40–45% 60% <		(Nastev et al., 2001)
11.	Increased nutrients in MSW	Y		(Christensen & Kjeldsen, 1989)

(*Continuted*)

TABLE 1.4 (Continued)

S.NO.	*PARAMETERS*	*INCREASE IN LFG GENERATION*	*DECREASE IN LFG GENERATION*	*REFERENCE*
12.	Increased microbial population	Y		(Malhotra & Mehta, 2002)
13.	High proportion of cellulose to lignin in MSW	Y		(Christensen & Kjeldsen, 1989)
14.	Increased oxygen in MSW		Y −200 mV −300 mV < 100 mV	(Christensen & Kjeldsen, 1989)
15.	Increased hydrogen in MSW		Y	(Barlaz et al., 1989)
16.	Increased sulphate content in MSW		Y	(Christensen & Kjeldsen, 1989)
17.	Toxicity of MSW		Y	(McCarty, 1964)
18.	Increased metals in MSW		Y	(Ehrig, 1983)
19.	Seeding of microorganisms	Y		(Eleazer et al., 1997)
20.	Buffer addition	Y		(Barlaz et al., 1989)
21.	Leachate recirculation	Y		(Reinhart et al., 2002)
22.	Rainfall/precipitation	Y		(Emcon Associates, 1980)
23.	Increase in atmospheric pressure		Y	(Poulsen et al., 2003)
24.	Increased porosity of landfill	Y 0.04 to 0.10		(El-Fadel & Rashed, 1998)
25.	Increased depth of MSW	Y		(El-Fadel & Rashed, 1998)
26.	Presence of high-permeability layers	Y		(Poulsen et al., 2001)
27.	Lower groundwater table	Y		(Nastev et al., 2001)
28.	Application of daily and final cover soil, impermeable liners	Y		(Nastev et al., 2001)

Note: Y: Yes

TABLE 1.5 Advances in LFG Potential

YEAR	*LFG POTENTIAL PER UNIT MSW*
2011	One tonne of MSW generates 442 m^3 of LFG (55% CH4). Around 12,200 m^3/day of LFG is generated per million tonnes of MSW. After the landfill is capped, the generation of LFG declines at 2%–15%/yr (Worrell & Vesilind, 2012).
2010	A rule of thumb for gas utilization (electricity generation) is that 1000 m^3/hr of LFG equals 1 MW of electricity generation.
2008	According to Long et al. (2008), 1 million tonnes of waste "in place" generate approximately 6 million m^3 of LFG per year. In 1 m^3 of LFG, there is approximately 0.357 kg of methane. Therefore, 1 million tonnes of MSW can generate around 2140 tonnes of CH4/year. Out of 2140 tonnes of generated methane, only 1500 tonnes can be recovered based on a collection efficiency of 70%.
2006	One tonne of waste can generate up to 150–200 m^3 of gas.
2004	Typically, LFG recovery rates may range between 25 and 100 m^3/hr for sites with MSW capacity of 100,000 m^3 and 250 to 10,000 m^3/hr or more for sites with capacities of 1–10 million m^3 (EA, 2004). 1.3 MW of power generation requires some 750 Nm^3/hr of LFG at 40–45 % CH4 concentration. To generate 1 MW of power, 700 Nm^3/hr of LFG (50% CH_4) is required.
2003	For the prediction of energy recovery from LFG, values ranging from 150–250 m^3/tonne are generally used. Typically, 600–700 m^3 of LFG (50% CH_4) is required to generate 1 MW of electricity (EPAI, 2003).
2002	One tonne of MSW will produce around 375 m^3 of LFG, with a calorific value (CV) of up to 20 MJ/m^3. A landfill containing 1 million tonnes of disposed MSW for over ten years will generate 700 m^3/hr methane at peak (Hester & Harrison, 2002).
2001	300 m^3 of LFG can be produced from 1 tonne of MSW. An average value is 4,75 kWh/m^3.
2000	One tonne of biodegradable waste can theoretically produce 400–500 m^3 LFG under optimized conditions. Typically, a value of 200 m^3 or less of LFG per wet tonne of MSW may be produced.

TABLE 1.6 Energy Content of LFG and Methane

S.NO.	*LFG ENERGY CONTENT (MJ/M^3)*	*METHANE ENERGY CONTENT (MJ/M^3)*	*REFERENCE*
1.	10, 13, 18	—	(Dace et al., 2015)
2.	19.7	—	(Worrell & Vesilind, 2012)
3.	20.5	—	(José et al., 2011)
4.	18–22	35.9	(Spokas et al., 2006)
5.	19	36	(Lappalainen & Kouvo, 2004)

TABLE 1.7 Categorization of Energy From Landfill Based on the Quality of LFG Recovered

LOW GRADE	*MEDIUM GRADE*	*HIGH GRADE*
• Removal of condensate or reduction in moisture content of LFG	• Compression as well as refrigeration along with chemical treatment such as scrubbing for removal of additional moisture content and LFG components present in trace amounts	• CO_2 separation and trace constituents from LFG and then compression to the desired limit
• Calorific value −16.8 MJ/m^3	• Calorific value −16.8 MJ/m^3	• Calorific value −37.3 MJ/m^3

1.3 LFG AND METHANE YIELD

1.3.1 LFG and Methane Yield Using Stoichiometric Method

Table 1.8 summarizes LFG and methane yield estimated by various researchers using the stoichiometric method.

It is observed from Table 1.8 that there is considerable variation in the estimates of LFG generation. Theoretical yields are generally higher, as they generally assume that all the biodegradable waste breaks down, but still there may exist pockets within a landfill where traces of decomposition occur due to lack of moisture content.

TABLE 1.8 LFG and Methane Yield Using Stoichiometric Method

S.NO.	TOTAL LFG YIELD (M^3/KG)	TOTAL METHANE YIELD (M^3/KG)	REFERENCE
1.	1.87	0.93	(Krause et al., 2016)
2.	—	0.415	(Cruz & Barlaz, 2010)
3.	—	0.581	(Worrell & Vesilind, 2012)
4.	—	0.342	(Worrell & Vesilind, 2012)
5.	—	0.436	(Themelis et al., 2007)

TABLE 1.9 LFG and Methane Yield Using Biodegradability Method

S.NO.	TOTAL LFG YIELD (M^3/KG)	TOTAL METHANE YIELD (M^3/KG)	REFERENCE
1.	0.13 (Dry)	0.19–0.27 (Dry)	(Blanchet, 1977)
2.	0.12	0.06	(Pacey, 1976)
3.	0.25 (Dry)	0.12 (Dry)	(Pfeffer, 1974)
4.	0.19 (Dry)	0.09 (Dry)	(Dair & Schwegler, 1974)
5.	0.19 (Dry)	0.047 (Dry)	(Schwegler, 1973)

1.3.2 LFG and Methane Yield Using Biodegradability Method

Table 1.9 summarizes LFG and methane yield estimated by various researchers using the biodegradability method.

The biodegradability method considers different biodegradation rates for various fractions of MSW. Net LFG generation can be represented as the sum of gases emitted by the decomposition of the individual waste fraction.

1.3.3 LFG and Methane Yield in Digester Studies

Table 1.10 summarizes LFG and methane yield estimated by various researchers in digester studies.

TABLE 1.10 LFG and Methane Yield in Digester Studies

S.NO.	*TOTAL LFG YIELD (M^3/KG)*	*TOTAL METHANE YIELD (M^3/KG)*	*REFERENCE*
1.	0.721–0.731	0.469	(Sridevi et al., 2015)
2.	—	0.23–0.37	(Fongsatitkul et al., 2012)
3.	0.70	—	(Bouallagui et al., 2005)
4.	0.45	0.32	(Bouallagui et al., 2004)
5.	0.514–0.695	0.257–0.451	(Bouallagui et al., 2003)

TABLE 1.11 LFG and Methane Yield in Laboratory Simulation/Full-Scale Studies

S.NO.	*TOTAL LFG YIELD (M^3/KG)*	*TOTAL METHANE YIELD (M^3/KG)*	*REFERENCE*
1.	—	0.272–0.294	(Behera et al., 2010)
2.	0.0092–0.0144	0.0003–0.00063	(Croft, 1991)
3.	—	0.077–0.107(Dry)	(Barlaz et al., 1989)
4.	0.068–0.163	0.0381–0.0925	(Pacey, 1989)
5.	—	0.047–0.097	(Barlaz et al., 1989)

1.3.4 LFG and Methane Yield in Laboratory Simulation/Full-Scale Studies

Table 1.11 summarizes LFG and methane yield estimated by various researchers in laboratory simulation/full-scale studies.

1.4 CONCLUSION

It is evident that the LFG has enough energy potential to meet the demands of a fairly high population around the globe. Several projects have been implemented and are currently operational to extract the potential. LFG and methane yield have been explored through on-site field projects and lab-scale and pilot plant studies. The studies discussed in this chapter report the total methane yield ranging between $0.00038-0.93\,m^3/kg$ and total LFG yield between $0.001-1.87\,m^3/kg$. The large range variation is observed due to technological advancements and the parameters used during the study, such as waste composition, temperature, and moisture condition.

REFERENCES

Barlaz, M. A., Schaefer, D. M., & Ham, R. K. (1989). Bacterial population development and chemical characteristics of refuse decomposition in a simulated sanitary landfill. *Applied and Environmental Microbiology*, *55*(1), 55–65. https://doi.org/10.1128/AEM.55.1.55-65.1989

Behera, S. K., Park, J. M., Kim, K. H., & Park, H. S. (2010). Methane production from food waste leachate in laboratory-scale simulated landfill. *Waste Management*, *30*(8–9), 1502–1508. https://doi.org/10.1016/J.WASMAN.2010.02.028

Blanchet, M. (1977). *Treatment and utilization of landfill gas: Mountain view project feasibility study*. . . Environmental Protection Agency, Office of Solid Waste.

Bouallagui, H., Ben Cheikh, R., Marouani, L., & Hamdi, M. (2003). Mesophilic biogas production from fruit and vegetable waste in a tubular digester. *Bioresource Technology*, *86*(1), 85–89. https://doi.org/10.1016/S0960-8524(02)00097-4

Bouallagui, H., Torrijos, M., Godon, J. J., Moletta, R., Ben Cheikh, R., Touhami, Y., Delgenes, J. P., & Hamdi, M. (2004). Two-phases anaerobic digestion of fruit and vegetable wastes: Bioreactors performance. *Biochemical Engineering Journal*, *21*(2), 193–197. https://doi.org/10.1016/J.BEJ.2004.05.001

Bouallagui, H., Touhami, Y., Cheikh, R., & Hamdi, M. (2005). Bioreactor performance in anaerobic digestion of fruit and vegetable wastes. *Process Biochemistry*, *40*(3–4), 989–995. https://doi.org/10.1016/j.procbio.2004.03.007

Buivid, M. G., Wise, D. L., Blanchet, M. J., Remedios, E. C., Jenkins, B. M., Boyd, W. F., & Pacey, J. G. (1981). Fuel gas enhancement by controlled landfilling of municipal solid waste. *Resources and Conservation*, *6*(1), 3–20. https://doi.org/10.1016/0166-3097(81)90003-1

Christensen, T. H., & Kjeldsen, P. (1989). Basic biochemical processes in landfills. In *Sanitary landfilling: Process, technology, and environmental impact* (pp. 29–49). Academic Press.

Croft, B. (1991). *Field-scale landfill gas enhancement. The Brogborough test cells*. Inst of Gas Technology, Chicago, Illinois, USA, 129–157.

Cruz, F. B. D. La, & Barlaz, M. A. (2010). Estimation of waste component-specific landfill decay rates using laboratory-scale decomposition data. *Environmental Science and Technology*, *44*(12), 4722–4728. https://doi.org/10.1021/es100240r

Dace, E., Blumberga, D., Kuplais, G., Bozko, L., Khabdullina, Z., & Khabdullin, A. (2015). Optimization of landfill gas use in municipal solid waste landfills in Latvia. *Energy Procedia*, *72*, 293–299. https://doi.org/10.1016/J.EGYPRO.2015.06.042

Dair, F., & Schwegler, R. (1974). Energy recovery from landfills. *Waste Age*, *5*(2).

Ehrig, H. (1983). Quality and quantity of sanitary landfill leachate. *Waste Management & Research*, *1*(1), 53–68. https://doi.org/10.1016/0734-242X(83)90024-1

Eleazer, W. E., Odle, W. S., Wang, Y. S., & Barlaz, M. A. (1997). Biodegradability of municipal solid waste components in laboratory- scale landfills. *Environmental Science and Technology*, *31*(3), 911–917. https://doi.org/10.1021/ES9606788

El-Fadel, M., Findikakis, A. N., & Leckie, J. O. (1996). Numerical modelling of generation and transport of gas and heat in landfills I. Model formulation. *Waste Management & Research: The Journal for a Sustainable Circular Economy*, *14*(5), 483–504. https://doi.org/10.1177/0734242X9601400506

El-Fadel, M., & Rashed, H. (1998). Settlement in municipal solid waste landfills: I. Field scale experiments. *The Journal of Solid Waste Technology and Management*, *25*(2), 89–98.

Emcon Associates. (1980). Methane generation and recovery from landfills. CRC Press, 1–139, ISBN: 0250403609.

EPAI (2003). *Landfill Manuals – Landfill Monitoring*, 2nd Edition, Environmental Protection Agency, Ireland.

Firmo, A. L. B., Guimarães, L. J. N., Maciel, F. J., & Juca, J. F. T. (2011). Estimate of Methane Generation in experimental landfill located at Muribeca landfill-Brazil using simplified methods. In Fourth International Workshop "Hydro-Physico-Mechanics of landfills", pp. 27–28.

Fischedick M., J. Roy, A. Abdel-Aziz, A. Acquaye, J.M. Allwood, J.-P. Ceron, Y. Geng, H. Kheshgi, A. Lanza, D. Perczyk, L. Price,E. Santalla, C. Sheinbaum, and K. Tanaka (2014). Industry. In: *Climate Change 2014: Mitigation of Climate Change. Contri-bution of Working Group III to the Fifth Assessment Report of the Intergovernmental Panel on Climate Change.* Cambridge University Press, Cambridge, United Kingdom, 739–810. http://www.ipcc.ch/report/ar5/wg3/

Fongsatitkul, P., Elefsiniotis, P., & Wareham, D. G. (2012). Two-phase anaerobic digestion of the organic fraction of municipal solid waste: Estimation of methane production. *Waste Management and Research*, *30*(7), 720–726. https://doi.org/10.1177/0734242X11429987

Gardner, N., & Probert, S. D. (1993). Forecasting landfill-gas yields. *Applied Energy*, *44*(2), 131–163. https://doi.org/10.1016/0306-2619(93)90058-W

Guzzone, B., & Leatherwood, C. (2007). Landfill gas use trends in the United States. *Biocycle*, *48*(9), 57.

Hester, R., & Harrison, R. (2002). *Environmental and health impact of solid waste management activities* (Vol. 18). Royal Society of Chemistry.

Kaza, S., Yao, L., Bhada-Tata, P., & Woerden, F. Van. (2018). *What a waste 2.0: A global snapshot of solid waste management to 2050.* World Bank Publications, 1–292, ISBN: 9781464813474.

Krause, M. J., Chickering, G. W., & Townsend, T. G. (2016). Translating landfill methane generation parameters among first-order decay models. *Journal of the Air and Waste Management Association*, *66*(11), 1084–1097. https://doi.org/10.1080/10962247.2016.1200158

Lappalainen, S., & Kouvo, P. (2004). *Evaluation of greenhouse gas emissions from landfills in the St. Petersburg area-utilization of methane in energy production*, METGAS. Publication-Northern Dimension Research Centre.

Long, Y., Guo, Q., Fang, C., Zhu, Y., & Shen, D. (2008). In situ nitrogen removal in phase-separate bioreactor landfill. *Bioresource Technology*, *99*(13), 5352–5361.

Malhotra, V., & Mehta, P. (2002). *High-performance, high-volume fly ash concrete: Materials, mixture proportioning, properties, construction practice, and case histories.* Supplementary Cementing Materials for Sustainable Development, 1–101, ISBN: 9780973150704.

Manfredi, S., Tonini, D., Christensen, T. H., & Scharff, H. (2009). Landfilling of waste: Accounting of greenhouse gases and global warming contributions. *Waste Management and Research*, *27*(8), 825–836. https://doi.org/10.1177/0734242X09348529

McCarty, L. P. (1964). Anaerobic waste treatment fundamentals, Part III, Toxic materials and their control. *Public Works*, *95*, 91–94.

Mondal, T., Choudhury, M., Kundu, D., Dutta, D., & Samanta, P. (2023). Landfill: An eclectic review on structure, reactions and remediation approach. *Waste Management*, *164*, 127–142. https://doi.org/10.1016/j.wasman.2023.03.034

Nastev, M., Therrien, R., Lefebvre, R., & Geélinas, P. (2001). Gas production and migration in landfills and geological materials. *Journal of Contaminant Hydrology*, *52*(1–4), 187–211. https://doi.org/10.1016/S0169-7722(01)00158-9

Pacey, J. (1976). Methane gas in landfills: Liability or asset. In *Proceedings of the fourth national congress on waste management technology, and resource and energy*. U.S. Environmental Protection Agency, pp. 168–190.

Pacey, J. O. H. N. (1989). Landfill design concepts in the United States. In *Sanitary landfilling: Process, technology, and environmental impact* (pp. 559–576). Academic Press.

Pfeffer, J. T. (1974). Temperature effects on anaerobic fermentation of domestic refuse. *Biotechnology and Bioengineering*, *16*(6), 771–787. https://doi.org/10.1002/BIT.260160607

Poulsen, T. G., Christophersen, M., Moldrup, P., & Kjeldsen, P. (2001). Modeling lateral gas transport in soil adjacent to old landfill. *Journal of Environmental Engineering*, *127*(2), 145–153. https://doi.org/10.1061/(ASCE)0733-9372(2001)127:2(145)

Poulsen, T. G., Christophersen, M., Moldrup, P., & Kjeldsen, P. (2003). Relating landfill gas emissions to atmospheric pressure using numerical modelling and state-space analysis. *Waste Management and Research*, *21*(4), 356–366. https://doi.org/10.1177/0734242X0302100408

Reinhart, D. R., McCreanor, P. T., & Townsend, T. (2002). The bioreactor landfill: Its status and future. *Waste Management and Research*, *20*(2), 172–186. https://doi.org/10.1177/0734242X0202000209

Rettenberger, G. & Stegmann, R. (1996). Landfill gas components. In *Landfilling of waste: Biogas*, Taylor & Francis, pp. 51–58.

Rueda-Avellaneda, J. F., Rivas-García, P., Gomez-Gonzalez, R., Benitez-Bravo, R., Botello-Álvarez, J. E., & Tututi-Avila, S. (2021). Current and prospective situation of municipal solid waste final disposal in Mexico: A spatio-temporal evaluation. *Renewable and Sustainable Energy Transition*, *1*, 100007. https://doi.org/10.1016/J.RSET.2021.100007

Schwegler, R.E. (1973). Energy recovery at the landfill. *Presented at the 11th Annual Seminar and Equipment Show of the Governmental Refuse Collection and Disposal Association*, Santa Cruz, California, November, 7–9.

Spokas, K., Bogner, J., Chanton, J. P., Morcet, M., Aran, C., Graff, C., Golvan, Y. M. Le, & Hebe, I. (2006). Methane mass balance at three landfill sites: What is the efficiency of capture by gas collection systems? *Waste Management*, *26*(5), 516–525. https://doi.org/10.1016/j.wasman.2005.07.021

Sridevi, V., Rema, T., & Srinivasan, S. (2015). Studies on biogas production from vegetable market wastes in a two-phase anaerobic reactor. *Clean Technologies and Environmental Policy*, *17*(6), 1689–1697. https://doi.org/10.1007/s10098-014-0883-8

Themelis, N. J., & Ulloa, P. A. (2007). Methane generation in landfills. *Elsevier*, *32*, 1243–1257. https://doi.org/10.1016/j.renene.2006.04.020

Tittlebaum, M. E. (1982). Organic carbon content stabilization through landfill leachate recirculation. *Journal* (Water Pollution Control Federation), *54*(5), 428–433.

UNEP. (2021). *Global assessment: Urgent steps must be taken to reduce methane emissions this decade*. https://www.unep.org/news-and-stories/press-release/global-assessment-urgent-steps-must-be-taken-reduce-methane

Worrell, W. A., & Vesilind, P. A. (2012). *Solid waste engineering* (2nd ed.). Cengage Learning.

Global Landfill Gas Emission Models

A Critical Analysis

2

Abdul Rafey, Faisal Zia Siddiqui, and Vasudevan Rajaram

2.1 INTRODUCTION

Globally, around 1.3 billion tonnes of municipal waste were produced in 2012, which rose to about 2.01 billion tonnes in 2018 (World Bank, 2018) and is projected to increase by 2025 to around 2.21 billion tonnes (Hoornweg & Bhada-Tata, 2012). Increasing industrialization, urbanization, rapid technological disruption, and changing life patterns accompany the process of economic growth, which will give rise to an entire generation of increasing quantities of waste that will invariably lead to increased environmental threats (Jha et al., 2008; Khajuria et al., 2010; Srivastava et al., 2014). Thus, with increased waste generation amounts, systematic management and safe handling have become areas of concern worldwide (Kumar et al., 2017). In most studies, landfill disposal is considered a common waste management practice globally (Nagendran et al., 2006; Mondal et al., 2023; Njoku et al., 2018). Yet management strategies have been started for recycling and reuse, and measures are being taken to decrease waste generation (Amini et al., 2012). The decomposition of organic waste in landfills emits landfill

DOI: 10.1201/9781003499695-2

gas (LFG), and it may be collected for use as an energy source, replacing fossil fuels (Manfredi et al., 2009). The methane (CH_4) concentration in LFG is around $50-55\%$, and carbon dioxide (CO_2) is $45-50\%$,with inorganic compounds contributing in traces (US EPA, 2020). The global warming potential (GWP) of CH_4 is 24 times that of CO_2 (IPCC, 2007). As LFG emissions increased over a decade, the GWP of CH_4 increased to 28–36 times as compared to CO_2. Thus, uncontrolled CH_4 emissions from landfills became a significant problem. In the USA, disposal in landfills is around 52% of the entire MSW produced (US EPA, 2019). Worldwide, 70% of CH_4 emissions are caused by human activities (e.g., landfill, agriculture, natural gas), of which 19.1% is attributed to LFG generation (Czepiel et al., 2003). The latest study shows that, globally, out of the total anthropogenic CH_4 emissions, $22-23\%$ are caused by waste disposal practices, thus making it the second-largest emission source (Scheutz et al., 2009). Landfill emissions decreased in industrialized countries and increased in developing countries (Agamuthu, 2013). As developing countries experience an increase in population, CH_4 emissions are projected to rise (IEA, 2009a, 2009b). Thus, CH_4 emissions mainly depend on the practices followed at landfill sites in different countries. Between 2005 and 2020, global CH_4 emissions from these landfills are predicted to increase by 9%. Primary sources of CH_4 emissions from MSW include the United States, Canada, China, Southeast Asia, and Russia (IEA, 2009a).

The US Environmental Protection Agency (EPA) estimated global CH_4 emissions from landfills in 2012 based on historical data from 1990 to 2030. The United States, China, Malaysia, Russia, and Mexico are the top countries that emit methane from MSW. Table 2.1 shows the landfill CH_4 emissions forecasts by region. These estimates were derived from a sequence of projections provided by countries when they became available and IPCC data sources of 2006.

Globally, CH_4 emissions from landfills were projected to have increased by nearly 12% between 1990 and 2005, from 706 to 794 $MtCO_2e$. Growing populations lead to more personal income, and expanding industry leads to

TABLE 2.1 Methane Emissions for MSW Landfills: 2010–2030 (MtCO2e) (US EPA, 2012)

COUNTRIES/REGIONS	*2010*	*2015*	*2020*	*2025*	*2030*
Countries with maximum emissions					
United States	130	128	128	128	128
Mexico	56	60	63	65	68
Russia	47	46	45	43	42
China	47	48	49	49	49
Malaysia	30	33	35	38	40

(Continuted)

TABLE 2.1 (Continued)

COUNTRIES/REGIONS	*2010*	*2015*	*2020*	*2025*	*2030*
Rest of the regions					
Asia	133	135	138	142	144
Africa	101	107	112	117	122
Europe	87	92	97	101	105
Central and South America	71	74	77	79	81
Middle East	67	72	77	82	86
Eurasia	56	59	62	64	67
North America	20	22	23	25	27
Total	**845**	**876**	**906**	**933**	**959**

increased waste output, both driving forces behind this trend. Between 2005 and 2030, emissions are expected to rise by nearly 21%, from 794 to 959 tonnes.

2.2 STANDARD PROTOCOL FOR LFG RECOVERY

An overview of methods used for measuring LFG from landfills is given in Table 2.2. Waste analysis and pumping trials are commonly used methodologies, as listed in Table 2.2 at S. Nos. 11 and 13.

2.2.1 Pump Test Methodology for a Typical Landfill

A pump test provides information on the available LFG volume and its quality in a typical landfill. The pump test methodology has the following objectives:

- During the extraction of LFG from the landfill, measure pressure/vacuum and LFG flow.
- To estimate the CH_4 levels of the LFG extracted during the pump test.
- To evaluate the lateral vacuum influence of the active pump test, measure the pressure/vacuum in the probes.

TABLE 2.2 Methodology for LFG Measurement From Landfills (Scharff et al., 2000)

S.NO.	*TECHNIQUE*	*PROCEDURE*
1.	Soil core measurement	In a laboratory, soil samples are obtained and incubated.
2.	Static closed chamber	Landfill receives a confined volume, and concentration of CH_4 is then measured.
3.	Dynamic closed chamber	To avoid methane build-up, an air flow is delivered through the chamber, similar to static closed chambers.
4.	Mass-balance method	CH_4 and CO_2 levels are measured at various heights surrounding a landfill.
5.	Micrometeorological method	Measuring gas flux densities above a landfill.
6.	Mobile plume measurement	Methane concentrations recorded across a transect screen in the downwind direction.
7.	Stationary plume measurement	Air samples are collected at predetermined sites around a landfill.
8.	Isotope measurement (methane oxidation)	Measuring the ratio of 12C/13C isotopes to determine quantitatively methane oxidation
9.	Sub-surface vertical gradient method	CH_4 emissions are determined by utilizing probes to measure CH_4 concentration gradients inside a landfill.
10.	Waste sampling from trial pits and boreholes	Observation/inspection of the nature of MSW to provide a qualitative assessment.
11.	Waste analysis	MSW samples are analysed chemically. LFG potential is indicated by volatile solids or organic carbon concentration. LFG can be generated using samples that are incubated in the lab.
12.	Measurement of passive LFG emissions	Measurement of LFG flow from boreholes or flux boxes in the landfill.
13.	Pumping trials	Pumping LFG from boreholes until a steady state is reached, with estimation of waste volume based on pressure decrease in the landfill.

- During the pump test, measure the air infiltration on the landfill surface by measuring the oxygen concentration of the extracted LFG.
- Refine the LFG recovery forecasts based on the pump test findings.

2.2.2 Static Testing of LFG

Static LFG testing aims to assess LFG recovery under baseline/static conditions. Therefore, the flow rate of LFG from the extraction well is monitored under atmospheric pressure without operating the blower and keeping the flow-controlling valves open at the inlet and outlet points of the test section. During static testing, all the key parameters are measured once the flow becomes stable.

2.2.3 Dynamic Testing of LFG

After static testing, a dynamic test is performed. The critical steps in Method 2E of USEPA for dynamic testing are as follows (USEPA, 2017):

Step 1: Measure initial static pressure at the primary extraction well;
Step 2: Set the vacuum pump at double the static pressure;
Step 3: Measure the CH_4 concentration and LFG flow rate in the main extraction well during this time;
Step 4: Monitor oxygen ingress in shallow pressure probes;
Step 5: Monitor any reduction in the initial static pressure in deep pressure probes to determine the ROI for a given gas well;
Step 6: Raise the rate of vacuum to four times the original static pressure, then repeat steps 3 to 5;
Step 7: Based on the outcomes in step 6, specifically the air infiltration, continue testing under an increased pumping rate.
Step 8: With the blower operation at the desired flow rate, the LFG probes (9 per well) must be monitored.

However, USEPA Method 2E can be modified for a landfill depending on the site conditions, such as

- If a constant flow rate is achieved within 1–2 hrs.
- Air ingress is monitored by measuring pressure at shallow probes (negative pressure is an indication of air ingress) and also by examining oxygen content in the extracted LFG ($O_2 > 10\%$ is an indication of air ingress).
- Measurements for pressure, LFG composition, and flow rate can be done on a morning and evening basis.

TABLE 2.3 Dynamic Testing Scenarios for LFG Measurement

S. NO.	*SCENARIO*	*REMARKS*
1.	High LFG flowrate with low methane concentration and air infiltration under vacuum	Suitable for unsecured landfills
2.	Medium LFG flowrate with high methane concentration and air infiltration under vacuum	May not be suitable for unsecured landfills
3.	Low LFG flowrate with high methane concentration and air infiltration under vacuum	May not be suitable for unsecured landfills
4.	High LFG flowrate with low methane concentration and without any air infiltration under vacuum	Suitable for sanitary landfills
5.	Medium LFG flowrate with high methane concentration and without any air infiltration under vacuum	Suitable for sanitary landfills
6.	Low LFG flowrate with high methane concentration and without any air infiltration under vacuum	Suitable for sanitary landfills

The various scenarios considered for dynamic testing of a landfill are given in Table 2.3.

2.2.4 LFG Well Adjustment Procedure

The purpose of LFG healthy field adjustment is to attain a steady state condition of the LFG collection system by stabilizing the flow and composition of LFG during extraction. The parameters such as methane, oxygen, and temperature are essential in healthy adjustment. The commonly used method for LFG flow adjustment is based on the flow of CH_4. As the LFG well flow increases, the LFG extraction rate ultimately becomes equal to the LFG generation rate within the radius of influence (ROI) of the well. This is the highest rate at which LFG can be recovered without introducing too much air inside the landfill. (Because the landfill isn't completely sealed, air infiltration will always be there, even when extracting at a lower rate than the LFG generation rate.) More air will be drawn into the landfill to compensate for the disparity between extraction and generation. Adding air to the landfill will limit future methane production by inhibiting anaerobic bacteria. Because of the non-uniformity of LFG extraction and the requirement to draw some air into the waste mass to regulate emission on the surface, it is critical to allow the air to enter the landfill to recover as much LFG as possible.

2.2.5 Monitoring of LFG Pressure Probes

LFG flows from high pressure or concentration to low pressure or concentration. Pressure probes aim to identify whether LFG has migrated beyond an established boundary. The probes are installed to measure LFG quality and static pressure at various distances from the main well. CH_4, O_2, balance gas, and pressure are all monitored. Atmospheric air is infiltrated into the landfill when the atmospheric pressure exceeds the landfill pressure. Pressure probes identify this. It is, therefore, important to monitor LFG migration through pressure probes.

2.2.6 Radius of Influence for Okhla Landfill

The ROI for a landfill can be estimated using the following formula:

$$Q_w = (K \times \pi \times R^2 \times t \times D \times r) / C$$

Rearranging this equation gives:

$$R = [(Q_w \times C)/(K \times \pi \times t \times D \times r)]^{1/2}$$

Where:

Q_W = Average well flow rate (L/sec).
K = Conversion factor, 1.157×10^{-8} (L/day)/(mL/sec).
R = Radius of influence (m).
t = Thickness of waste (m).
D = Average bulk density of waste (kg/m^3).
r = Rate of CH_4 production (mL/kg/day).
C = Fractional methane concentration under dynamic conditions.
Q_{LFG} = Flow rate of LFG for entire landfill.
CCH_4 = Percent of methane in LFG under static conditions.
V_{MSW} = Volume of MSW disposed in the landfill.

2.3 COMMERCIAL APPLICATIONS OF LFG

- LFG energy projects transforms landfill gas into usable energy source suitable for variety of applications. The generation of power or usage as transportation fuel can be brought about by LFG.

- LFG can be used straight away or converted into pipeline-quality natural gas.
- LFG can be used directly for onsite leachate evaporation to evade leachate collection and treatment system costs.
- LFG can directly used in boilers instead of natural gas, coal, or fuel oil.
- Other potential uses include cogeneration, that is, combining heat and power production.
- Direct thermal applications, such as infrared heaters, dryers, and pottery kilns, can benefit from LFG.
- Other novel applications include lighting, heating greenhouses, and heating water for aquaculture operations.
- LFG is currently used in various industries, including the automobile sector, chemical sector, food processing sector, pharmaceutical sector, cement sector and brick kiln production, effluent treatment, electronics sector, pulp and paper sector, and steel sector, including hospitals.
- LFG may be converted to natural gas by purification methods since its composition is comparable to that of natural gas.

2.4 MODEL PARAMETERS FOR LFG PREDICTION

The development of equations or computer-based models that form the basis for estimating the CH_4 production rate relies heavily on baseline/primary and secondary data. Limited parameters would result in more erroneous results compared to on-site field research. On the other hand, more complicated and detailed parameter involvement results in more accurate projection. Different mathematical models account for the projection of various parameters; however, model outputs are subject to high uncertainty due to inadequate projection or a lack of data (Amini et al., 2012). The following section presents different baseline and secondary parameters required for LFG prediction.

2.4.1 Baseline Parameters for LFG Prediction

Baseline parameters required for LFG prediction are mass of waste; lag time; slowly and rapidly decomposable waste fraction; age of waste; biodegradable organic fraction; time for the start of methane generation and peak rate time;

moisture content; landfill design capacity; conversion time; content of organic carbon in waste; landfill opening and closing year; daily, intermediate and final cover material surface area and property; percentage coverage; seasonal methane oxidation in each cover type; distribution of waste type; and aerobic/ anaerobic conditions.

2.4.2 Secondary Parameters for LFG Prediction

Secondary parameters required for LFG prediction include methane generation potential, rate constant, decay rate, first-order rise phase constant, rate of decay for slowly and rapidly decomposable waste, concentration of total and non-methane organic compounds (NMOCs), dissimilation factor, conversion factor, adsorptive capacity, leachate head, waste density, hydraulic conductivity, porosity, normalization factor, percent biodegradable carbon, percent biodegradable carbon converted, the collection efficiency of the LFG recovery system, methane concentration, history of landfill fires, gas collection efficiency, discount factor for fire, annual waste disposal rate, average annual precipitation, decay half-life, methane correction factor, and half-life time of solid waste.

2.5 GLOBAL LFG MODELS

The first-order kinetic model is the most popular model for LFG generation modelling compared to zero- and second-order models. Research on the zero-order model concludes that the outcomes are inconsistent due to high inaccuracy levels, but inaccuracy in higher-order models is slightly lower (Govindan & Agamuthu, 2014). As one progresses from a first- to a second-order method, the modelling procedure increases in complexity, but a gain in accuracy does not accompany this; hence most of the LFG models are developed using first-order kinetics (Oonk et al., 1994). Table 2.4 shows the order of various LFG models.

TABLE 2.4 Classification of Global LFG Models Based on Their Order

S.NO.	*NAME OF MODEL*	*YEAR OF MODEL*	*ORDER OF MODEL*
1.	Zero order	1987	0
2.	Triangular	1993	0
3.	EPER model Germany	2001	0

S.NO.	*NAME OF MODEL*	*YEAR OF MODEL*	*ORDER OF MODEL*
4.	First order	1976–2010	1
5.	Scholl Canyon	1976	1
6.	Sheldon Arleta	1976	1
7.	Palos Verdes	1977	1
8.	EMCON MGM	1983	1
9.	Tabasaran model	1987	1
10.	Modified first order	1994	1
11.	GASFILL	1988	Two phase
12.	LFGGEN	1994	1
13.	TNO	1994	1
14.	IGNiG model	1994	1
15.	Multiphase model	1995	1 exponential
16.	Multiphase model (Afvalzorg)	1996, 2011, 2012, 2014	1
17.	LandGEM (version 2.0, 3.02, 3.03)	1998, 2005, 2020	1
18.	RET screen model (v1.0, v4.0, Plus, Suite, Expert, Expert v8.0)	1998, 2007, 2011, 2012, 2016, 2020	1
19.	EPER model France	2001	1, multiphase
20.	GasSim (v1.0, v2.0, v2.5)	2002, 2006, 2012	1, multiphase
21.	Mexico model (v1.0, v2.0)	2003, 2009	1
22.	IPCC model	1996, 2006	1
23.	Central America model	2007	1
24.	Philippines model	2009	1
25.	Thailand model	2009	1
26.	Ukraine model	2009	1
27.	China model	2009	1
28.	Ecuador model	2009	1
29.	Colombia model	2010	1
30.	Second order	1994	2
31.	CALMIM model	2011	Field validated

2.6 RESEARCH GAPS IN THE DEVELOPED LFG MODELS

Different drawbacks in existing LFG models are presented in Table 2.5.

TABLE 2.5 Drawbacks in Existing Global LFG Models

S.NO.	*MODEL*	*DRAWBACKS*
1.	Multiphase model	For various waste categories, detailed information on carbon content and its quality is required.
2.	Scholl Canyon	Lag phase is assumed to be negligible. Moisture content not accounted for.
3.	Stoichiometric	Provides assessment of total LFG generated and not generation rate. Non-biodegradable waste fractions such as lignin and plastics are not stoichiometrically estimated. Moisture content is not accounted for.
4.	Triangular	Moisture content is not accounted.
5.	Palos Verdes	For individual waste category, methane potential is not considered. Inaccurate supposition that one-half of LFG is generated in every phase.
6.	Sheldon Arleta	Assumption that at peak rate half of LFG is generated is inaccurate.
7.	LandGEM	Inappropriate for countries with different climatic conditions or different mix of wastes. Range of default k values is limited and no guidance on appropriate k values for countries experiencing higher precipitation rates.
8.	TNO	In order to anticipate LFG generation on other sites, the values of the composition of waste have been fixed in the model.
9.	Multiphase model (Afvalzorg)	For some of the waste types, there is a lack of data on organic matter/carbon content.
10.	EPER model France	The normalization factor has been considered in the model equation but not accounted for in the spreadsheet. The dimensionality of the multiphase equation for LFG generation is insufficient.

S.NO.	MODEL	DRAWBACKS
11.	EPER model Germany	Only household or comparable waste type is considered.
12.	CALMIM model	The model does not explicitly project LFG generation, but it does take into account the landfill components that control emissions. It also considers additional gaseous transport processes besides diffusion, as well as the physical features of compacted soil.
13.	IPCC model	Does not take into account consequences of higher precipitation rates such as those exceeding 1000 mm.year^{-1}. Because precipitation has a bigger impact on LFG formation than temperature, they should not be weighted equally in climate models. Potential evapotranspiration (PET) is yet to be validated for many locations, and there is no data on PET, so it should not be used to assign climate in temperate areas.
14.	Finite-element model	Model involves prediction of LFG generation through coupled partial differential equations by breaking the landfill into tiny elements, but model could not be validated with real-time data.
15.	Tabasaran model	The model accounts for the duration of sludge retention in a biodigester operating under anaerobic conditions. The temperature correction factor in projecting LFG generation potential is not suitable for landfills.

2.7 CONCLUSIONS

LFG is important due to its uncontrolled emission to the atmosphere, contributing to being a key source of GHG. Therefore, an accurate model for predicting LFG generation and recovery from a landfill plays a key role in LFG management of any region or country. Although the LFG modelling option has been well exploited by developed countries, it is yet to be established fully as a viable option for effective waste management in developing countries. Thus, for a complete solution of waste management, structured LFG modelling has to be applied, which takes into account all options and gives the best possible option for solid waste management based on local conditions and waste scenarios.

REFERENCES

Agamuthu, P. (2013). Landfilling in developing countries. *Waste Management and Research*, *31*(1), 1–2. https://doi.org/10.1177/0734242X12469169

Amini, H. R., Reinhart, D. R., & Mackie, K. R. (2012). Determination of first-order landfill gas modeling parameters and uncertainties. *Waste Management*, *32*, 305–316. https://www.sciencedirect.com/science/article/pii/S0956053X11004272

Czepiel, P. M., Shorter, J. H., Mosher, B., Allwine, E., McManus, J. B., Harriss, R. C., Kolb, C. E., & Lamb, B. K. (2003). The influence of atmospheric pressure on landfill methane emissions. *Waste Management*, *23*(7), 593–598. https://doi.org/10.1016/S0956-053X(03)00103-X

Govindan, S. S., & Agamuthu, P. (2014). Quantification of landfill methane using modified Intergovernmental Panel on Climate Change's waste model and error function analysis. *Waste Management and Research*, *32*(10), 1005–1014. https://doi.org/10.1177/0734242X14552551

Hoornweg, D., & Bhada-Tata, P. (2012). What a waste: A global review of solid waste management. *The World Bank*, *15*, 1–116. https://doi.org/10.1201/9781315593173-4

IEA. (2009a). *Energy sector methane recovery and use* International Energy Agency, Paris, p. 46.

IEA. (2009b, January 28). *Turning a liability into an asset: The importance of policy in fostering landfill gas use worldwide*. https://www.iea.org/publications/freepublications/publication/landfill.pdf

IPCC. (2007). *Climate change 2007—Synthesis report* (p. 112). https://doi.org/10.1038/446727a

Jha, A. K., Sharma, C., Singh, N., Ramesh, R., Purvaja, R., & Gupta, P. K. (2008). Greenhouse gas emissions from municipal solid waste management in Indian mega-cities: A case study of Chennai landfill sites. *Chemosphere*, *71*(4), 750–758. https://doi.org/10.1016/j.chemosphere.2007.10.024

Khajuria, A., Yamamoto, Y., & Morioka, T. (2010). Estimation of municipal solid waste generation and landfill area in Asian developing countries. *Journal of Environmental Biology*, *31*(5), 649–654.

Kumar, S., Smith, S. R., Fowler, G., Velis, C., Kumar, S. J., Arya, S., Rena, Kumar, R., & Cheeseman, C. (2017). Challenges and opportunities associated with waste management in India. *Royal Society Open Science*, *4*(3). Royal Society. https://doi.org/10.1098/rsos.160764

Manfredi, S., Tonini, D., Christensen, T. H., & Scharff, H. (2009). Landfilling of waste: Accounting of greenhouse gases and global warming contributions. *Waste Management and Research*, *27*(8), 825–836. https://doi.org/10.1177/0734242X09348529

Mondal, T., Choudhury, M., Kundu, D., Dutta, D., & Samanta, P. (2023). Landfill: An eclectic review on structure, reactions and remediation approach. *Waste Management*, *164*, 127–142. https://doi.org/10.1016/j.wasman.2023.03.034

Nagendran, R., Selvam, A., Joseph, K., & Chiemchaisri, C. (2006). Phytoremediation and rehabilitation of municipal solid waste landfills and dumpsites: A brief review. *Waste Management*, *26*(12), 1357–1369. https://doi.org/10.1016/j.wasman.2006.05.003

Njoku, P. O., Odiyo, J. O., Durowoju, O. S., & Edokpayi, J. N. (2018). A review of landfill gas generation and utilisation in Africa. *Open Environmental Sciences*, *10*(1), 1–15. https://doi.org/10.2174/1876325101810010001

Oonk, H., Weenk, A., Coops, O., & Luning, L. (1994). Validation of landfill gas formation models. *NOVEM Programme Energy Generation from Waste and Biomass (EWAB)*, TNO report, 94–315, Apeldoorn, Netherlands.

Scharff, H., Oonk, J., Hensen, A., (2000). Quantifying landfill gas emissions in the Netherlands– Definition study. *NOVEM Programme Reduction of Other Greenhouse Gases (ROB)*, project number 374399/9020, Utrecht, Netherlands. http://www.robklimaat.nl/ docs/3743999020.pdf

Scheutz, C., Kjeldsen, P., Bogner, J. E., De Visscher, A., Gebert, J., Hilger, H. A., Huber-Humer, M., & Spokas, K. (2009). Microbial methane oxidation processes and technologies for mitigation of landfill gas emissions. *Waste Management and Research*, *27*(5), 409–455. https://doi.org/10.1177/0734242X09339325

Srivastava, V., Ismail, S. A., Singh, P., & Singh, R. P. (2015). Urban solid waste management in the developing world with emphasis on India: Challenges and opportunities. *Reviews in Environmental Science and Biotechnology*, *14*(2), 317–337. https://doi.org/10.1007/s11157-014-9352-4

US EPA (2012). Global anthropogenic non-CO_2 greenhouse gas emissions: 1990–2030. *U.S. Environmental Protection Agency*, Washington. https://www.epa.gov/global-mitigation-non-co2-greenhouse-gases/global-non-co2-ghg-emissions-1990-2030

US EPA (2017). Method 2E: Determination of landfill gas production flow rate. *U.S. Environmental Protection Agency, Washington*. https://www.epa.gov/sites/default/files/2017-08/documents/method_2e.pdf

U.S. EPA. (2019, November). Advancing sustainable materials management: 2017 Fact Sheet. *United States environmental protection agency* (p. 22). https://www.epa.gov/facts-and-figures-about-materials-waste-and-recycling/advancing-sustainable-materials-management%0Ahttps://www.epa.gov/smm/advancing-sustainable-materials-management-facts-and-figures-report

U.S. EPA. (2020, March). *LFG energy project development handbook* (p. 139). https://www.epa.gov/sites/production/files/2016-07/documents/pdf_full.pdf

World Bank. (2018, September 23). *World Bank: Global waste generation could increase 70% by 2050 | Waste Dive*. https://www.wastedive.com/news/world-bank-global-waste-generation-2050/533031/

Waste to Energy

A Case Study of Christ University, India

3

Vikas Janardhan Salunkhe and Sarangapani Nivarthi

3.1 INTRODUCTION

Rapid economic growth paved the way for increased living standards, resource consumption, and the quantity and complexity of waste generation. Per the data published by the World Bank (*What a Waste: An Updated Look Into the Future of Solid Waste Management*, 2018), approximately 2.01 billion tons of solid waste is generated worldwide every year. According to this report, around 33% of the waste is not being managed in an environmentally friendly manner, which is one reason for the impact of climate change. A study by the World Bank in 2018 the inevitable rise in urbanization, marginal population growth, and related developments around the globe will contribute to a 70% increase in waste over the next 30 years. The lack of sophisticated waste treatment and management in hazardous industrial, nuclear, and biomedical wastes is prone to amplifying environmental and health-related issues. In many countries, improper management of biomedical waste is transporting pathogens, while industrial wastes like oils, discarded paints, and chemicals are causing significant adverse impacts on human health

DOI: 10.1201/9781003499695-3

and the environment. To mitigate the adverse effects of an increase in different forms of waste on the environment and average life of humans, waste is now regarded as a resource rather than an unwanted thing. Reduce, reuse, and recycle philosophies are now acting as alternatives to waste management. Efficient utilization of available resources and minimization of wastes will reduce the cost of operation of business entities and also provide several upstream benefits like lower susceptibility to unreliable materials, reduced reliance on global markets for critical materials, and reduced depletion of natural resources. As an integral part of society, higher education institutions also undertake many initiatives for sustainable development. Many higher education institutions are adopting innovative practices toward waste management on their campuses. Christ University is one such university contributing towards this through a centre called the Centre for Social Action and Parivarthana. Per the Sustainable Development Goals (SDGs), each goal is scientifically interlinked; therefore, adequate emphasis should be given to all the goals to achieve the desired target. Chetana is a sustained child-focused development project, an independent registered body under the Karnataka Souharda Co-operative Societies Act. Christ University has committed itself to contributing to achieving the goals through various activities.

- Sustainable Development Goal 1: Self-help groups and child sponsorship for underprivileged children.
- Sustainable Development Goal 2: Around 100+ students from ongoing Centre for Social Action projects receive free lunch at Christ University every year. During this pandemic time, 300 food packets were distributed at various places per day and continued.
- Sustainable Development Goal 3: Free health check-ups like Reverse Transcription Polymerase Chain Reaction (RT PCR). Free Coronavirus Disease 2019 (COVID-19) doses. Outreach by Centre for Counselling and Health Services (CCHS) at campus.
- Sustainable Development Goal 4: Students at ongoing Centre for Social Action projects in various states of India are provided education free of cost.
- Sustainable Development Goal 5: Equal opportunity for all.
- Sustainable Development Goal 6: Waste and sewage water treatment. Reuse of recycled water.
- Sustainable Development Goal 7: Production of biogas through waste food. Solar panels. Use of LEDs.
- Sustainable Development Goal 8: Community Development Programs. Slum area development. Self-help groups. Donations from the recycling unit.
- Sustainable Development Goal 9: Infrastructure development, inclusive and sustainable industrialization promotion, and innovative ideas.

- Sustainable Development Goal 10: The Child Sponsorship Programme of the Centre for Social Action extends to children from various marginalized groups; it also includes some children from denotified and nomadic communities.
- Sustainable Development Goal 11: To make the lives of humans and other living organisms sustainable. The faculty and students have been involved in providing sustainable solutions and have helped foster sustainable cities.
- Sustainable Development Goal 12: Reuse, recycle, and reproduction out of waste.
- Sustainable Development Goal 13: To achieve the target of net-zero waste and sustainable development, environmental-friendly waste management is the best way.
- Sustainable Development Goal 14: Aquaculture is yet to be implemented.
- Sustainable Development Goal 15: Gardening, 100% organic vegetable production.
- Sustainable Development Goal 16: The Vision and Mission of Christ University, Excellence and Service to All, is being served in all aspects of teaching, learning, research, and community engagement.
- Sustainable Development Goal 17: The goal targets energizing and reinvigorating a strategy of implementing the desired goals in terms of a global partnership for sustainable development. The university has partnered with several governmental, non-governmental, and corporate entities in the country and globally.

3.2 WASTE MANAGEMENT IN HIGHER EDUCATIONAL INSTITUTIONS

Educational institutions are leading in shaping young minds to contribute to managing societal waste. The University of Oxford responsibly focuses on waste management at its campus to mitigate waste generation. Stakeholders at the University of Oxford are opting for the best ways to alleviate waste production in the first place: reuse and recycle. The great endeavour of 24,000 students and 13,600 staff members is to be well aware of the waste they generate and put their minds to different ways to alleviate waste generation. The Faculty of Civil Engineering and Planning at the Islamic University of Indonesia has evaluated solid waste management on campus using the "zero waste index" (Iresha et al., 2018). The recent outbreak of COVID-19 resulted in the mass production of medical products, for instance, masks, PPE, testing kits, hand gloves, helmets, and related materials (Choudhury et al., 2022). Inoculation has generated massive amounts of medicinal waste. Teaching hospitals affiliated with Isfahan University of Medical Sciences conducted an awareness program for nurses on medical waste management in 2014, which can be a model at present to tackle the issue of medical waste (Iresha et al., 2018).

Harvard University has six ways to minimize e-waste, with the strong belief that minimizing e-waste will help conserve resources and reduce the energy we acquire from the earth: re-evaluating, improving the life of electronic gadgets, procuring environmentally friendly electronics, gifting used electronics to marginalized strata of society in social programs, re-using big electronics, and recycling electronics and batteries in e-waste recycling bins across the university. St John's College, and University of Cambridge, has a policy on waste management for 2021 that certainly focuses on waste segregation and recycling on campus. The involvement of stakeholders, such as housekeeping and management, includes crystal clear regulations on the collection and use of waste generated at the University of Cambridge. Challenging issues related to waste management require the attention of agencies working in the field of not-for-profits, governments, and social activists. The role of anthropology in waste management has been explained for laypersons by Patric O'Hare, University of Cambridge (Alexander & O'Hare, 2020).

The Massachusetts Institute of Technology (MIT), designing waste and contamination, is continuously endeavouring in rigorous ways, with the various departments, science labs, material scientists, and behavioural researchers, to reduce the generation of waste and convert it into clean material for reuse purposes (e.g., paper waste, food waste, and plastics). The strategies being followed at MIT are reducing, promoting, growing, developing, evaluating, and testing waste. University College London has a new year's resolution: working towards a greener and more sustainable campus. Tony Overbury, lead of waste management, estates, and facilities, responsible for managing waste generated at the campus, provides some prioritized suggestions. He emphasizes not procuring unnecessary stuff. In a simple way, he is asking necessary questions to reduce unnecessary procurement, such as: Do I need it? Do I need packaging? Can I reuse it? Can I recycle it? And where can I find out more? (2008). The California Institute of Technology follows a unique way of collecting e-waste on campus. The safety office at Caltech collects e-waste, including batteries, cassette players, computers, copiers, keyboards, laptops, printers, scanners, monitors, and mobile phones. At Imperial College London, they prioritize how to reuse and recycle the waste generated on campus. Conservation of natural resources, saving energy, protecting the environment, and mitigating the waste going to the landfill are all important goals. Priority has been given to reusing rather than recycling, recycling rather than incineration, and recovering energy rather than just burning waste, which are policies to ensure valuable waste has not been wasted and does not contribute to landfills. Imperial College London recently sent a significant amount of waste to recover energy from landfills. The University of Chicago is managing all hazardous waste per regulations set up by the federal, state, and local authorities. Careful identification and labelling of all waste containers, maintaining a proper schedule for waste pick-up, avoiding waste piling, ensuring waste segregation, adhering to legitimized rules and regulations while disposing of hazardous waste, and conducting periodic audits are essential practices.

The University Grant Commission (2017), which coordinates higher education institutions (HEIs) in India, has given guidelines to ban plastic on campus and maintain zero-waste and green campuses (2017). The guidelines say that the government of India has decided to make the plastic ban a national-level campaign to address the environmental hazards and bring about attitudinal changes that shun the use of plastics. The various stages of solid waste management involve waste segregation, collection, and transportation from the initial point of the source of waste to recycling and disposal at the destination point (Talsania & Modi, n.d.). The 3R strategy of reduce, re-use, and re-produce has been implemented in various higher education institutions in India to encourage waste management. The complexity of recycling and reusing waste materials is triggered by the heterogeneous nature of the waste created (Pappu et al., 2007). Moreira et al. (2018) present the Solid Waste Management Index (SWaMI) implemented in three different universities in Brazil and one in the US and statistically compare the results to give specific strategies for policy makers regarding waste management in HEIs.

Municipal solid waste (MSW) from educational institutions (Jayaprakash & Jagadeesan, 2019) includes various elements such as vegetable waste, food scraps, packaging, paper, plastic, and more. These facilities produce about 500 kg of garbage daily and 8,000 kg of paper and cardboard monthly. Costs associated with disposal, clogged drains, vector breeding, and contaminated soil are among the main issues. Proper waste management (Jayaprakash & Jagadeesan, 2019) is essential to minimize waste generation and maximize value-added products. Food, plastics, and packaging materials are among the many types of municipal solid waste that educational facilities produce (Felder et al., 2001). Some of the main issues are soil contamination, drain obstruction, vector breeding, and disposal expenses. The University of British Columbia commissioned a solid waste audit in 1998 to ascertain residual trash characteristics and offer reduction guidance. Facilities with distinct collection systems for tracking user traffic and seasonal trash are best suited for the audit technique (Felder et al., 2001). In response to student concerns about environmental management, a university campus implemented a zero-waste program (Mason et al., 2003). The program included working group meetings, funding proposals, externally sponsored research programs, and interactions with academic and local government workers. Senior management's written policy and dedication to environmental responsibility served as support.

The MIT Office of Sustainability aims to enhance the recycling of clean materials such as paper, plastics, and food waste while decreasing the amount of trash produced on campus (n.d.) through partnerships with various departments, labs, and researchers. Decreases in emissions, pollution, and waste recovery are the objectives (n.d.). Promoting the reuse of single-use items, developing an online market for surplus materials, acquiring materials from renewable sources, taking the material's life cycle into account, and evaluating waste management techniques are some of the tactics.

3.3 WASTE MANAGEMENT IN CHRIST UNIVERSITY: A ROADMAP FOR SUSTAINABILITY

As higher education institutions gather momentum in their influence on graduate lives, it is increasingly important to make the learning journey of young citizens holistic. Along these lines, Christ University realizes the significance of respect for nature in and around the campus, ensuring that students and other stakeholders play their part as responsible citizens.

Christ University established an exclusive unit called Centre for Social Action in 1999 to address issues related to marginalized community development; child rights; socio-economic development of women, youth, and farmers; and environment or climate change. To overcome these issues and extend community services, the institution started venturing into a campus waste management unit named Parivarthana to *transform* waste into wealth. Parivarthana is the decentralized waste management unit of Christ University with the guiding motto of Reduce, Reuse, and Recycle. It was established in 2008. This unit covers various functions like manure or compost production, sewage water treatment, paper recycling, biogas, nursery (gardening), zero waste or waste reduction at source, and rainwater harvesting. Its core objective is "To maintain the status of Christ University as a 'Zero Waste Campus' by reusing and recycling the maximum waste generated here".

3.4 SOURCES OF WASTE GENERATION AT CHRIST UNIVERSITY

Around 1000 to 1200 kg of waste is generated at Christ University due to day-to-day activities. Approximately 25,000+ stakeholders at Christ University generate waste through regular activities like consumption of food and water;

use of study materials and chemicals in the laboratory; and use or disposal of electronic equipment like computers, laptops, mobile, various scientific instruments, and other related items. Other waste includes food waste, sewage water, used papers, pens, DVDs, CDs, pen drives, telescopes, observation equipment, air conditioning machines, electric and electronic waste, solar panels, tree leaves, used furniture, materials used for co-curricular and extracurricular activities, and clothes used in theatre or cultural activities.

3.5 COLLECTION OF WASTE

Dustbins are placed with proper labelling at every corner of the campus, like dry and wet waste (Moladoost et al., 2016). Awareness signboards encourage students to separate waste properly, ensuring that most of the waste gets separated at the source. The dedicated housekeeping staff of the university, with the help of waste collection vehicles, collects waste from the bins and dumps it at the storehouse of the Parivarthana Unit. Segregation at the source is the principle.

3.6 SEGREGATION OF WASTE

This procedure is followed to segregate the waste collected at the university. The designated staff divides most of the waste from bins labelled "Dry Waste, Wet Waste" placed at every corner of the university. At the recycling unit, they divide the waste into different categories like e-waste, paper waste, tree leaves, solid waste, food waste, tetra packs, electric and electronic waste, glass waste, hazardous waste, and others. Most importantly, the waste that will not be recycled or composted is stored separately and handed over to the Municipal Corporation.

3.7 PROCESS OF WASTE MANAGEMENT

The waste that is collected is processed in the following ways:

- **Tree leaves:** Tree leaves and other related waste are sent to the compost unit.

- **Tetra packs:** Collected tetra packs are distributed among the common interest groups (CIGs) located in slum areas in and around Bengaluru. Members of the CIGs produce handbags and other related durable and eco-friendly products. Samples are shown subsequently.
- **Food waste** is divided into two categories, cooked and raw. Cooked waste is sent to the biogas plant, and raw waste is sent to the compost generation unit for clean energy and manure as output products, respectively.
- **Paper waste:** All the waste from student activities and administrative offices is recycled and converted into office files, pen stands, photo frames, paper pens, posters, flyers, greeting cards, and many more, as shown subsequently.
- **Hazardous waste:** Hazardous waste like chemicals from the science lab, batteries from the physics lab, preserves from the bio lab, broken glass, and other related waste is being stored carefully and transported to the Municipal Corporation Bengaluru for recycling purposes or otherwise.
- **Sewage water:** Through the underground network of drainage lines, wastewater is collected and sent to the water treatment plant. After that, treated water is used for the garden and flushed in the toilets.

3.8 OUTCOMES POST-RECYCLING AND REPRODUCTION; BENEFICIARIES AND COMMUNITY INVOLVEMENT

The following are the outcomes of recycling and reproduction:

Paper products: Two or four times a month, social work and sociology students set up a stall to sell paper products. The total revenue is donated to marginalized groups in the slum areas and other community development projects maintained by the Centre for Social Action (Salunkhe, n.d.). One prominent child development program is the 3D Empowerment Project (Desirable, Dynamic, and Development). A portion of the revenue is used for 3D projects, too.

- **Manure:** Pesticide-free and environmentally friendly tonic for trees.
- **Food waste:** Approximately 25 kgs/ day biogas.
- **Recycled water:** To maintain greenery in and around the university, garden, plantation, and nursery.
- **Others:** 100% organic vegetables and fruits like mango, tamarind, banana, and berry. A variety of beautiful flowers.

The beneficiaries of the initiative include

- **Individuals:** Each and every stakeholder of the university.
- **Society and community:** Subjects involved in the related projects.
- **Environment/climate change:** Pollution-free environment.
- **Living organisms:** Herbivores in and around the campus.

Community involvement and employment generation: Through the self help groups (SHGs) and common interest groups, Christ University contributes to employment generation. Not only educated but also illiterate individuals can sustain themselves with the various community-centric initiatives of Christ University.

3.9 THE META PICTURE

The Centre for Social Action (CSA) and Parivarthana have left an impactful impression in and around Christ University and on society.

- **Conservation of energy:** Waste to energy through the production of biogas.
- **Net zero waste:** Through converting waste into compost or manure.
- **Recycling:** Recycling paper waste and reproducing paper products, considering the conservation of natural resources like trees, water, and energy.
- **Nation development:** The heterogeneous initiatives of Christ University in the areas of rural development, community organizations, land development, and agricultural development in the various states of India like Karnataka, Kerala, Telangana, Maharashtra, and Chhattisgarh.

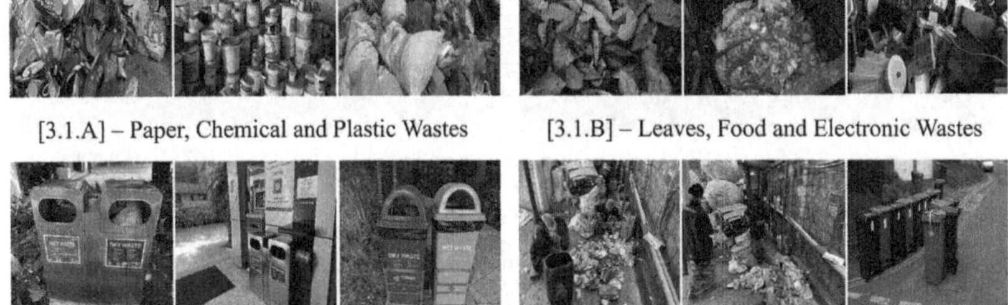

[3.1.A] – Paper, Chemical and Plastic Wastes

[3.1.B] – Leaves, Food and Electronic Wastes

[3.1.C] – Collection, Segregation and Storage of Wastes

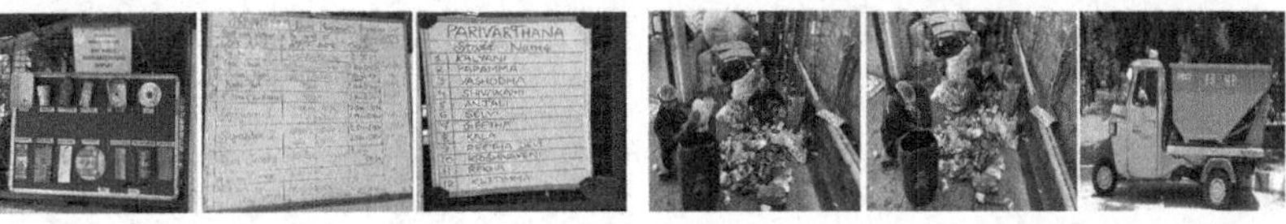

[3.1.D] – Segregation Display Board, Collection Spots, and Responsible Staff Members

[3.1.E] – Storage and Segregation Area, and Municipal Corporation Vehicle

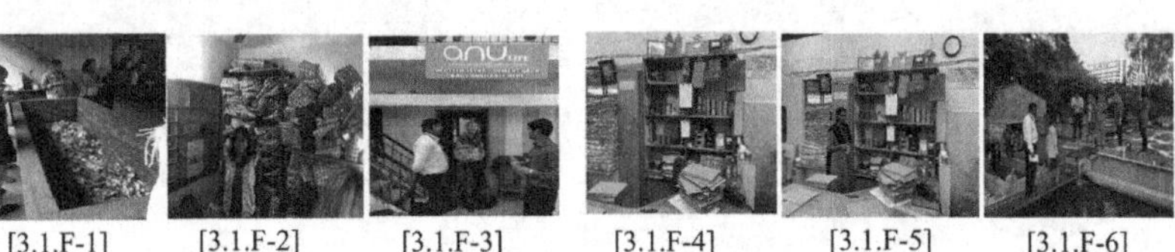

[3.1.F-1] [3.1.F-2] [3.1.F-3] [3.1.F-4] [3.1.F-5] [3.1.F-6]

[3.1.F] – (1) Visit of Griffith University Australia to Compost Unit. (2) Handbags made of Tetra Packs. (3) ANU Life – A New Life out of Wastes, shop in slum area supported by CSA.

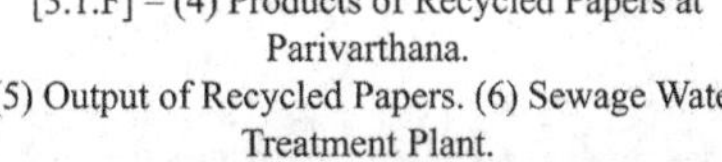

[3.1.F] – (4) Products of Recycled Papers at Parivarthana.
(5) Output of Recycled Papers. (6) Sewage Water Treatment Plant.

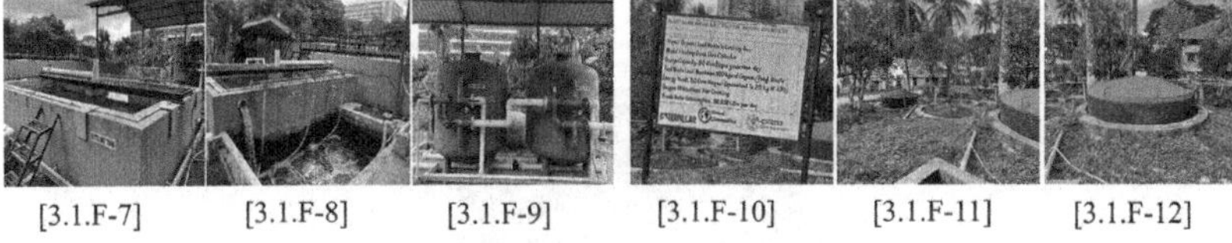

[3.1.F-7] [3.1.F-8] [3.1.F-9] [3.1.F-10] [3.1.F-11] [3.1.F-12]

[3.1.F] – (7) Sewage Treatment Plant. (8) Sewage Treatment Plant. (9) Recycled Water Purification.

[3.1.F] – (10) Biogas Plant Banner. (11) Biogas Plant. (12) Biogas Plant - Unit.

Christ University, Bangalore, Karnataka, India. Parivarthana (Recycling Unit – Paper and Water Recycling)

FIGURE 3.1 (a) Paper, chemical, and plastic wastes. (b) Leaves, food, and electronic wastes. (c) Collection, segregation, and storage of wastes. (d) Segregation display boards, collection spots and responsible staff. (e) Store, segregation area, and municipal corporation vehicle. (f) (1) Visit of Griffith University, Australia, to the compost unit. (2) Handbags made of tetra packs. (3) ANU Life—A New Life out of Wastes, shop in slum area supported by CSA. (4) Products of recycled paper at Parivarthana. (5) Output of recycled papers. (6–8) Sewage water treatment plant. (9) Recycled purified water. (10) Biogas plant signboard. (11) Biogas plant. (12) Biogas plant–unit.

[3.2.A] – Stall at Campus
[3.2.B] – Ready Manure
[3.2.C] – Nursery
[3.2.D] – Campus Beautification

[3.2.E] – Campus Beautification
[3.2.F] – Recycled Water Storage
[3.2.G] – 100% Organic Vegetables

Christ University, Bangalore, Karnataka, India. Parivarthana (Recycling Unit – Outcome-Based Applications)

[3.2.H] – Parivarthana Office and Staff
[3.2.I] – Greenery on Campus
[3.2.J] – Self Help Group - Hoskote
[3.2.K] – School at Hoskote

[3.2.L] – Community at Hoskote
[3.2.M] – 3D Project in Slum Janakiramnagar Bangalore
[3.2.N] – Oxidation of Recycled Water
[3.2.O] – Community Managed Resource Centre – Hoskote, Bangalore

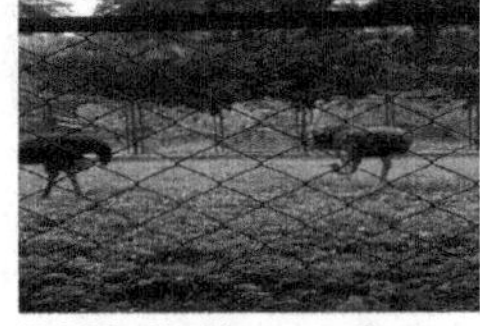

[3.2.P] – Herbivores on Campus

Christ University, Bangalore, Karnataka, India. Parivarthana (Recycling Unit – Ongoing Projects in Slum and Rural Areas)

FIGURE 3.2 (a) Stall on campus. (b) Ready manure. (c) Nursery. (d–e) Campus beautification. (f) Recycled water storage. (g) 100% organic vegetables. (h) Parivarthana Office and Staff. (i) Greenery on campus. (j) Self-help group—Hoskote. (k) School at Hoskote. (l) Community at Hoskote. (m) 3D Project in slum Janakiramnagar, Bangalore. (n) Oxidation of recycled water. (o) Community-managed resource centre—Hoskote, Bangalore. (p) Herbivores on campus.

3.10 CONCLUSION

Environmental protection and sustainability are the responsibilities of every individual, institution, corporate entity, and society, including higher education institutions. Many HEIs contribute to them by employing sustainable practices in their campuses. Creating awareness and engaging the community in several sustainable practices improve the level of sustainability of the institutions, too. Waste management is one of the areas in which sustainability can be ensured and community (students, staff, and researchers) engagement can be taken care of. To provide a more holistic perspective, higher educational institutions need to drive society through sustainable development. In this regard, many universities are working to achieve sustainable development goals. In this chapter, an attempt is made to highlight such higher education institutions. Also, a case study on sustainable practices followed by Christ University, India, on waste treatment and management is done. Through the Centre for Social Action and Parivarthana, the university has initiated many activities like manure or compost production, sewage water treatment, paper recycling, biogas, nursery (gardening), zero waste or waste reduction at the source, rainwater harvesting, and so on. The sole objective of these initiatives is to achieve sustainable development goals by ensuring that students and other stakeholders play their role as responsible citizens in nation-building in particular and the sustainable world at large.

ACKNOWLEDGEMENTS

The authors would like to thank Dr. Fr Joseph Varghese, director, Centre for Research and Publication, Christ University, India. He is also a professor, Dept. of Mathematics, Christ University, India. We appreciate the guidance and support throughout our endeavour in this regard.

REFERENCES

Alexander, C., & O'Hare, P. (2020). Waste and its disguises: Technologies of (un)knowing. *Journal of Anthropology*, *88*(3), 419–443. https://doi.org/10.1080/00141844.2020.1796734

Choudhury, M., Sahoo, S., Samanta, P., Tiwari, A., Tiwari, A., Chadha, U., Bhardwaj, P., Nalluri, A., Eticha, O. K., & Chakravorty, A. (2022). COVID-19: An accelerator for global plastic consumption and its implications. *Journal of Environmental and Public Health, 2022*, 17. https://doi.org/10.1155/2022/1066350

Felder, M. A., Petrell, R. J., & Duff, S. J. (2001). A solid waste audit and directions for waste reduction at the University of British Columbia, Canada. *Waste Management & Research: The Journal for a Sustainable Circular Economy*, *19*(4), 354–365. https://journals.sagepub.com/doi/10.1177/0734242X0101900412

Iresha, F. M., Prasojo, S. A., & Kasam, K. (2018). Evaluation of solid waste management at campus using the “Zero Waste Index”: The case on campus of Islamic University of Indonesia. *Earth and Environmental Sciences*, *154*(02004), 5. https://www.matec-conferences.org/articles/matecconf/abs/2018/13/matecconf_icet4sd2018_02004/matecconf_icet4sd2018_02004.html

Jayaprakash, J., & Jagadeesan, H. (2019). Sustainable waste management in higher education institutions—a case study in AC Tech, Anna University, Chennai, India. *Green Engineering for Campus Sustainability*, *1*, 163–172. https://link.springer.com/chapter/10.1007/978-981-13-7260-5_12#citeas

Mason, I. G., Brooking, A. K., Oberender, A., Harford, J. M., & Horsley, P. (2003). Implementation of a zero waste program at a university campus. *Resources, Conservation and Recycling*, *38*(4), 257–269. https://doi.org/10.1016/S0921-3449(02)00147-7

Moladoost, A., Farzi, S., & Shirazi, M. (2016). Sedigheh Farzi Sedigheh Farzi Nurses’ awareness of medical waste management in teaching hospitals affiliated to Isfahan University of Medical Sciences at 2014. *Iran Journal of Nursing*, *29*(99), 66–75. https://scholar.google.com/citations?view_op=view_citation&hl=en&user=or_wkRYAAAAJ&citation_for_view=or_wkRYAAAAJ:zYLM7Y9cAGgC

Moreira, R., Malheiros, T. F., Alfaro, J. F., Cetrulo, T. B., & Ávila, L. V. (2018). Solid waste management index for Brazilian Higher Education Institutions. *Waste Management*, *80*, 292–298. https://doi.org/10.1016/j.wasman.2018.09.025

Pappu, A., Saxena, M., & Asolekar, S. R. (2007). Solid wastes generation in India and their recycling potential in building materials. *Building and Environment*, *42*(6), 2311–2320. https://doi.org/10.1016/j.buildenv.2006.04.015

Salunkhe, V. J. (n.d.). *Community involvement and employment generation*. Christ University.

Talsania, P., & Modi, N. (n.d.). A review of waste generation, characterisation and solid waste management practices using bottoms-up approach in educational buildings. *International Journal of Research and Analytical Reviews*, *6*(2), 866–869. http://ijrar.com/upload_issue/ijrar_issue_20543639.pdf

University Grants Commission. (2017, November 9). *Swachhata Hi Sewa Campaign*. YouTube: Home. Retrieved January 28, 2024, from https://www.ugc.ac.in/pdfnews/8170476_UGC-Guidelines-for-Ban-of-Plastic-Use-in-%20%20%20%20%20%20%20%20Higher-%20Education-Institutions.p

Waste | MIT Sustainability. (n.d.). MIT Office of Sustainability. Retrieved January 28, 2024, from https://sustainability.mit.edu/tab/waste

What a waste: An updated look into the future of solid waste management. (2018, September 20). World Bank. Retrieved January 28, 2024, from https://www.worldbank.org/en/news/immersive-story/2018/09/20/what-a-waste-an-updated-look-into-the-future-of-solid-waste-management

Population Dynamics of Gamma Proteobacteria 4

Critical Analysis during Different Phases of Composting

Sutripta Sarkar, Rajdeep Banerjee, Sunanda Chanda, Sandipan Ganguly, and Pradeep Das

4.1 INTRODUCTION

Composting, being a biological process, involves a myriad of microorganisms. The microorganisms, composition, and magnitude are important components of the composting process. A study of the inherent microbial population is important to understand the composting process. The conversion of organic

DOI: 10.1201/9781003499695-4

material during composting depends on the inherent microbes and their activities (Paul et al., 2019). Classical measurement methods of microbiological activity in composts involve determining and enumerating the number of mesophilic and thermophilic microorganisms present. However, culturable counts do not give a clear picture of the microbial community, as it represent the population that can grow in the conditions provided for cultivation (Sarkar et al., 2010). It is not a true representative of the microbial communities actually present in the system. Direct microscopy reveals a cell count that may exceed the number of colonies derived from plating by several orders of magnitude (Smaruj & Bocian, 2020). Some of these "missing cells" might not be viable, but many microorganisms cannot be cultured on the standard media used to determine viable counts. Others may, in principle, be culturable but occur in a physiological state where the cells are viable but nonculturable (Wideman et al., 2021). Cell viability might be judged by morphological changes or changes in membrane permeability and/or physiological state inferred from the exclusion of certain dyes or the uptake and retention of others (Wideman et al., 2021). The LIVE/DEAD Baclight viability kit (Molecular Probes Inc., Eugene, Oregon) differentiates live and dead bacteria based on plasma membrane permeability. It contains two dyes, SYTO9 and propidium iodide (PI). SYTO 9 (excitation and emission maxima, 480 and nm) penetrates both viable and nonviable bacteria. In contrast, propidium iodide (excitation and emission maxima, 490 and 635 nm) only penetrates bacteria with damaged plasma membranes, quenching the green STYO 9 fluorescence. Thus, bacterial cells with compromised membranes fluoresce red, and those with intact membranes fluoresce green.

New technologies have led to a better estimation of microbial communities and their physiological role in ecosystems. In situ identification of individual microbial cells with fluorescently labelled, rRNA-targeted oligonucleotide probes is widely used due to their ability to estimate many microbes in any environmental system. Flow cytometry is an extremely versatile tool that complements existing technologies and enables fundamentally new information to be obtained in microbial ecology studies (Ancona et al., 2014; Hong et al., 2021; Di Lenola et al., 2020). Around 3,000 – 100,000 cells per second can be characterized and sorted by a flow cytometer. Microbial cells can be distinguished based on size, shape, surface texture, viability, and DNA content (Edwards, 2020). Flow cytometry has been used in the enumeration of bacteria in activated sludge (Brown et al., 2019), water treatment (Rockey et al., 2019), milk (Li et al., 2021) and hydrothermal vent (Parikka et al., 2018). In Composting systems, the studies of Diaper and Edwards (1994) and Sarkar et al. (2010), used flow cytometric data for community compost analysis. Several other researchers have also recently used flow cytometry to study microbial community dynamics (Shin et al., 2009; Yoon et al., 2013; Narihiro et al., 2016). A study by Piceno et al. (2017) highlighted the community shift in thermophilically treated human waste. The hybridized cells were viewed by a confocal microscope in the current study for a better assessment. This study was undertaken to understand the population dynamics of class γ-proteobacteria bacteria. This study is significant because proteobacteria is one of the most abundant phyla present during composting (Vivas et al., 2009), and γ- proteobacteria is the most profuse and physiologically diverse sub-group among proteobacteria.

4.2 MATERIALS AND METHODS

4.2.1 Field Setup

All field trials were carried out at Gupta Niwas (ISI farm) between the months of November and April. The proportion of vegetable waste, rice straw and dung was 5 : 1 : 0.2. Leafy vegetable waste was collected from the market and air dried for 48 h. The composting pile was set up as mentioned by Sarkar et al. (2016). Temperature change, moisture content, CN ratio and pH were monitored regularly. Samples were collected on days 0, 1, 2, 3, 4 and 15 and stored at –70°C for microbial and biochemical studies.

4.2.2 Biochemical Estimations

The biochemical analysis methods followed were as given in Sarkar et al. (2016). The percentage of organic carbon (total) was estimated by the Walkley and Black method (1934) and nitrogen by the Kjeldahl method (Association of Analytical Chemists (AOAC), 1984).

4.2.3 Determination of pH

An air-dried compost sample (10 gms) was taken in a 250-ml beaker containing 50 ml distilled water. After rigorously stirring and allowing the solid particles to settle down, the pH of the suspension was read with a pre-calibrated pH meter (Systronics Model no. 802).

4.2.4 Determination of Moisture Content (dry wt.)

Ten grams of compost sample (wet weight) was weighed in a glass petri dish (initial wt.) and dried in an oven set at 105°C until a constant weight (final weight) was reached. Final weight subtracted from initial weight gave the moisture content.

4.2.5 Fluorescence In Situ Hybridization

To probe γ- Proteobacteria, an oligonucleotide complementary to the 23S rRNA sequence of *E. coli* between nucleotide positions 1027 and 1043 (GCCTTCCCACATCGTTT) (GAMv 42a) was used (Siyambalapitiya & Blackall, 2005). The probe was labelled with fluorescein isothiocyanate (FITC) by Gibco BRL. One g of compost sample was fixed overnight in 3 ml of 4% paraformaldehyde solution (prepared in Phosphate Buffer Saline (PBS). Fixed samples were centrifuged and washed in PBS.

For hybridization reactions a buffer was used having the following composition -20 mM Tris-HCl pH 7.2; 0.9 M sodium chloride; 0.1% SDS. The washed cells were suspended in 100μl hybridization buffer (prewarmed at 48°C) in Eppendorf tubes; 2 ng/μl of FITC tagged γ- proteobacterial probe was added, and cells were hybridized at 48°C for 2h. After hybridization, cells were washed thrice in the hybridization buffer at 46°C and centrifuged. The hybridized cells were then enumerated by flow cytometer and observed under the confocal microscope. *E. coli* was kept in positive control, and *Geobacillus stearothermophilus* was kept as negative control. Unhybridized cells from compost were kept blank.

4.2.6 Confocal Microscope

The stained cells were taken in a slide and viewed under a confocal microscope LSM 510 meta (Carl Zeiss Ltd.). Randomly selected areas of each sample were imaged using a v 100X magnification objective with a numerical aperture 1.4 . Confocal illumination was provided by an argon laser (488 nm laser excitation) fitted with a long-pass 514 nm emission filter. A c 580 -nm beam splitter was used with a long-pass 515 nm filter (green fluorescence signal) and a long-pass filter 560 nm (red fluorescence signal). Simultaneous dual-channel imaging using pseudocolour displayed green and red fluorescence. The confocal pinhole was set at 1. Red-green images were acquired using zoom factor 1.

4.2.7 Sample Preparation for Live-Dead Cell Count

Bacterial live-dead cytometric count (Cytomics FC 500) was performed by Live-Dead Baclight bacterial viability and counting kit (LIVE/DEAD Baclight bacterial viability kit, Molecular Probes, Eugene, USA) per the manufacturer's instructions. The ratio of a number of reference microspheres to the number of cells detected by the cytometer gave the cell count. WINMDI 2.9 software was used to analyse the data (Sarkar et al., 2010).

4.2.8 Statistical Analysis

All results shown are a mean of three replicates. Analysis was carried out using SPSS and Microsoft Excel.

4.3 RESULTS AND DISCUSSION

Due to the intense microbial activity, an increase in temperature was observed after 24 h on day 1. The temperature shot up to 66°C on day 1, and then it further increased to 69.5°C on day 2. The temperature gradually decreased to 42.5°C on day 15. The thermophilic phase lasted for over 15 days (Figure 4.1a). Three phases were distinctive during the decomposition process: (a) mesophilic phase (below 40°C), (b) thermophilic phase (above 40°C) and (c) cooling or maturation phase. The effect of temperature on the composting process and its microbial inhabitants has been studied by several workers (Strom, 1985; Ishii et al., 2000; Sarkar et al., 2010). However, this still intrigues researchers, as the high temperature is one of the extreme environmental stresses to which organisms are exposed, requiring many molecular adaptations for tolerance and growth (Merino et al., 2019). Temperature is also a fundamental factor affecting the rate and net outcome of chemical and biochemical reactions (Johnson et al., 1974). In piles of sufficient size, organic-rich matter tends to heat up as the inherent microbial community breaks down the utilizable substrate, producing metabolic heat which, when trapped, can elevate the temperature of the pile to 70°C or above (Moreno et al., 2021). Such a habitat provides a unique opportunity to study the succession of diverse microbial communities about changing temperature over relatively short periods of time (Moreno et al., 2021). A decline in the C/N ratio was observed during the study, indicating the conversion of complex carbon into

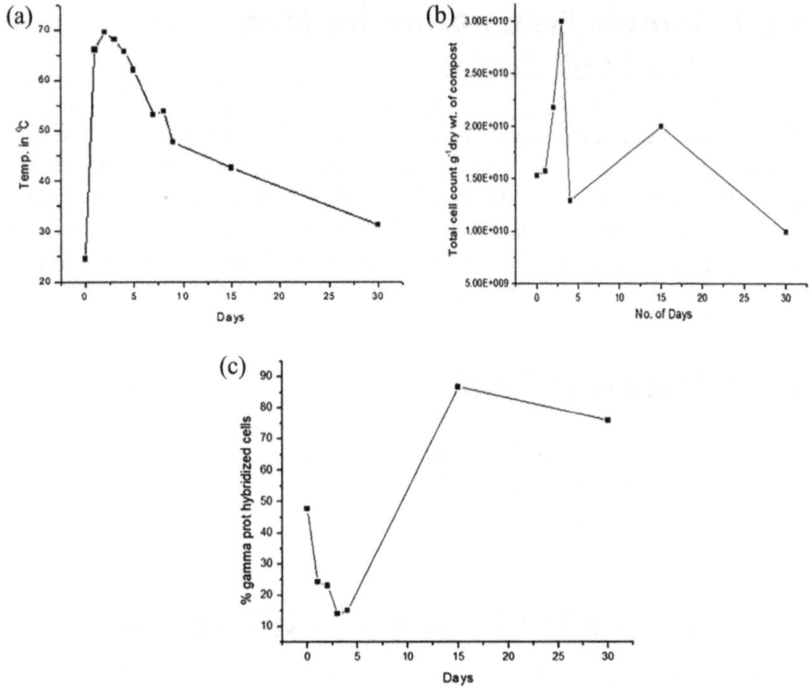

FIGURE 4.1 (a) Change in temperature during composting. (b) Change in total (live+dead) cell count during composting. (c) Percentage change in hybridized cells with γ-proteobacterial probe.

carbon dioxide (Table 4.1). The physicochemical parameters were found to be similar to previous studies (Sarkar et al., 2016), indicating that the composting process was well standardized. The carbon content of compostable material decreased with time, and nitrogen content per unit of material increased, resulting in the decreased C/N ratio (Goyal et al., 2005). Many studies report a high count of thermophilic bacteria during the heating phase (Ryckeboer et al., 2003). Temperatures close to 70°C (Strom, 1985) and the raw materials used might not have supported the growth of mesophilic bacteria.

With the increase in temperature, the total cell count (live + dead cells) increased, and the maximum count was recorded on day 3. Confocal micrographs of live-dead are shown in Figure 4.2(a) and 4.2(b). There was a decrease in total count on day 4 (Figure 4.1(b)), which might have been due to the prolonged high temperatures hurting cell growth (Ryckeboer et al., 2003).

Different day compost samples were hybridized by γ- proteobacterial probe, and the number of cells hybridized was counted by flow cytometer

TABLE 4.1 Physico-Chemical Characteristics of Compost

SAMPLING DAYS	*TEMPERATURE (°C)*	*PH*	*% MOISTURE CONTENT*	*C/N RATIO*
Day 0	24.5	7.16	67.56	15.1
Day 1	66.0	7.20	68.65	13.8
Day 2	69.5	7.9	70.73	12.9
Day 3	68.0	8.1	73.62	11.5
Day 4	65.7	8.2	70.77	10.2
Day 15	42.5	8.2	64.15	6.95
Day 30	31.3	7.9	57.5	5.8

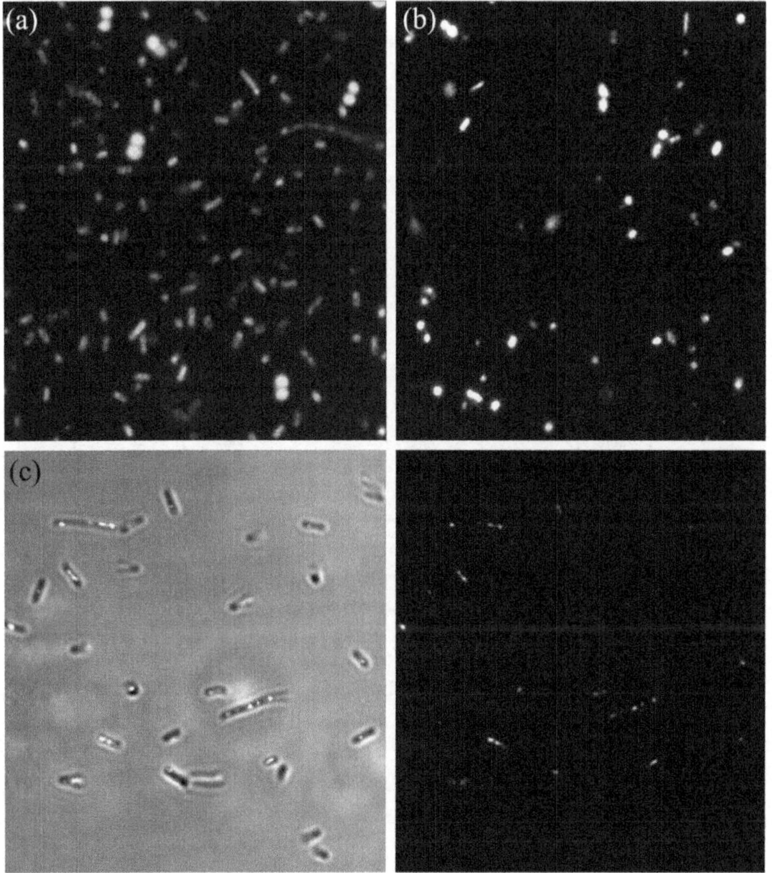

FIGURE 4.2 (a) Confocal micrograph showing live + dead *Escherichia coli*. (b) Confocal micrograph showing live + dead compost samples. (c) Confocal micrograph showing hybridized γ proteobacteria in compost samples.

(Figure 4.3(a–j)), which revealed the change in percentage population of γ- proteobacteria through different phases of composting (Figure 4.1(c)). A high count of γ- proteobacteria was observed during the initial stages of composting. Initial hybridization was 47%, which is comparable to 52% γ- proteobacterial cells, reported by Takebayashi et al. (2007).

However, their numbers decreased during the thermophilic phase, and again, an increase was observed in the cooling and maturation phase. A strong negative correlation ($R^2 = -0.87$) was observed between temperature and percentage

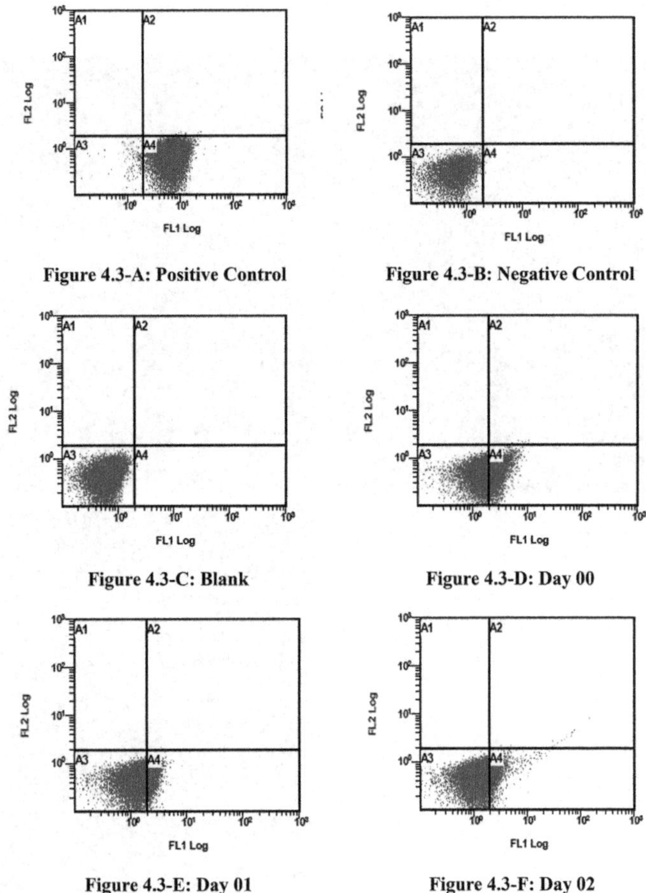

FIGURE 4.3 The cytograms depict the shift in population of γ- proteobacteria cells during composting. (a) *E.coli* cells hybridized with the γ- proteobacterial probe. (b) *G. stearothermophilus* cells hybridized with the γ- proteobacterial probe. (c) unhybridized compost sample. (d–j) Compost samples collected on different days hybridized with γ- proteobacterial probe.

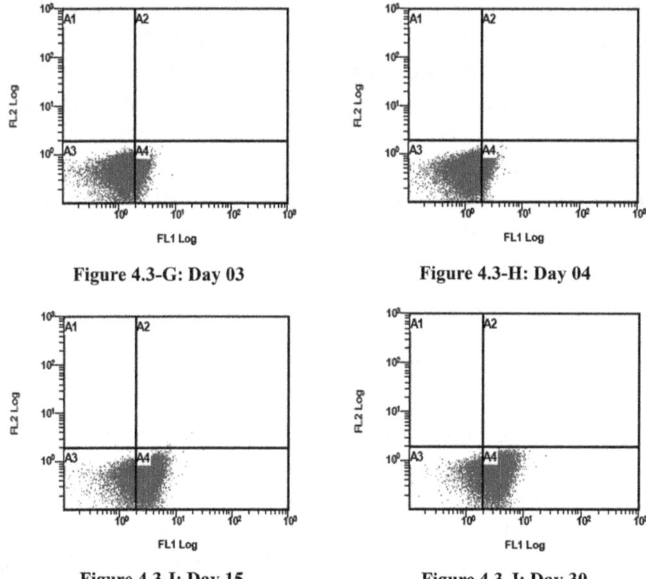

Figure 4.3-G: Day 03

Figure 4.3-H: Day 04

Figure 4.3-I: Day 15

Figure 4.3-J: Day 30

FIGURE 4.3 (Continued)

population of γ- proteobacteria. This indicates that most of the members of the subgroup of γ- proteobacteria were mesophiles, and high temperatures proved derogatory for their growth. It has been reported by earlier workers (Strom, 1985; Takaku et al., 2006) that *Bacillus* sp. dominates the thermophilic phase of composting. However, few have reported the fate of bacteria belonging to the class γ- proteobacteria, which is also quite dominant during composting (Ishii et al., 2000). Takaku et al. (2006) reported an increase in the population of γ-proteobacteria in the cooling and maturation phase, which is like the results we obtained. Danon et al. (2008) also reported γ- proteobacteria to be the most populous organism during the curing phase of composting. A confocal micrograph showing hybridized cells in a compost sample is given later (Figure 4.2(c)).

This study is significant because proteobacteria are one of the most abundant phyla present during composting (Vivas et al., 2009), and γ- proteobacteria is the most profuse and physiologically diverse subgroup among proteobacteria. Research shows that proteobacteria predominates initial composting, and there is a shift towards Actinobacteria and Firmicutes in the later phases. Change in water availability leads to a shift in population (Takebayashi et al., 2007), and changes in temperature profile during composting lead to changes in microbial population dynamics (Takaku et al., 2006; Tang et al., 2007). Hiraishi et al. (2003) reported a similar shift in microbial populations during flowerpot-using solid biowaste composting (FUSBIC) processes. Takaku et al. (2006) used the

Denaturing Gradient Gel Electrophoresis (DGGE) method for microbial community profiling, and Tang et al. (2007) used quinone profiling to determine the community structure. Flow cytometric methods allow a more thorough characterization of microbial communities than microbial cultivation or the methods mentioned previously; hence, they have been used for enumeration and characterization of microbial communities in activated sludge (Brown et al., 2022). To the best of our knowledge, this is the first systematic study on the fate of γ- proteobacteria during the various phases of composting using flow cytometry.

CONCLUSION

Compost is one of the most complicated biosystems. The process of biodegradation and the role of the microbial communities involved have intrigued researchers for a long time. The advent of modern technology in ecological studies has not only helped to develop clearer perceptions of microbial structures and dynamics but also has opened a lot of new avenues for research. This chapter is a step towards unravelling the simple yet less understood microbial world.

ACKNOWLEDGEMENTS

The authors thank the director, Indian Statistical Institute, Kolkata, and the principal of Barrackpore Rastraguru Surendranath College for their support.

REFERENCES

Ancona, V., Barra Caracciolo, A., Grenni, P., Di Lenola, M., Calabrese, A., Campanale, C., & Felice Uricchio, V. (2014, May). Microbiological indicators for assessing ecosystem soil quality and changes in it at degraded sites treated with compost. In *Geophysical Research Abstracts* Vol. 16 (p. 15215).

AOAC. (1984). In W. Horwitz (Ed.), *Official Methods of Analysis, 14*(p. 1141). Association of Official Analytical Chemists, Washington, DC, p. 1141.

Brown, M. R., Hands, C. L., Coello-Garcia, T., Sani, B. S., Ott, A. I. G., Smith, S. J., & Davenport, R. J. (2019). A flow cytometry method for bacterial quantification and biomass estimates in activated sludge. *Journal of Microbiological Methods, 160*, 73–83.

Brown, P., Ikuma, K., & Ong, S.K. (2022). Biological phosphorus removal and its microbial community in a modified full-scale activated sludge system under dry and wet weather dynamics. *Water Research, 217*, 118338.

Danon, M., Frank-Whittle, I. H., Insam, H., Chen, Y., & Hadar, Y. (2008). Molecular analysis of bacterial community succession during prolonged compost curing. *FEMS Microbiology Ecology*, *65*, 133–144.

Diaper, J. P., & Edwards, C. (1994). Flow cytometric detection of viable bacteria in compost. *FEMS Microbiology Ecology*, *14*, 213–220.

Di Lenola, M., Barra Caracciolo, A., Ancona, V., Laudicina, V. A., Garbini, G. L., Mascolo, G., & Grenni, P. (2020). Combined effects of compost and medicago sativa in recovery a PCB contaminated soil. *Water*, *12*(3), 860.

Edwards, C. (2020). Assessment of viability of bacteria by flow cytometry. In *Flow cytometry applications in cell culture* (pp. 291–310). CRC Press.

Goyal, S., Dhull, S. K., & Kapoor, K. K. (2005). Chemical and biological changes during composting of different organic wastes and assessment of compost maturity. *Bioresource Technology*, *96*, 1584–1591.

Hiraishi, A., Narihiro, T., & Yamanaka, Y. (2003). Microbial community dynamics during start-up operation of flowerpot-using fed-batch reactors for composting of household biowaste. *Environmental Microbiology*, *5*, 765–776.

Hong, J. K., Kim, S. B., Ahn, S. H., Choi, Y., & Lee, T. K. (2021). Flow cytometric monitoring of the bacterial phenotypic diversity in aquatic ecosystems. *Journal of Microbiology*, *59*(10), 879–885.

Ishii, K., Fukui, M., & Takii, S. (2000). Microbial succession during a composting process as evaluated by denaturing gradient gel electrophoresis analysis. *Journal of Applied Microbiology*, *89*, 768–777.

Johnson, F.H., Eyring, H., & Stover, B.J. (1974). *The theory of rate processes in biology and medicine*. John Wiley and Sons INC., New York.

Li, F., Santillan-Urquiza, E., Cronin, U., O'Meara, E., McCarthy, W., Hogan, S.A., Wilkinson, M.G., & Tobin, J.T. (2021). Assessment of the response of indigenous microflora and inoculated Bacillus licheniformis endospores in reconstituted skim milk to microwave and conventional heating systems by flow cytometry. *Journal of Dairy Science, 104*(9), 9627–9644.

Merino, N., Aronson, H. S., Bojanova, D. P., Feyhl-Buska, J., Wong, M. L., Zhang, S., & Giovannelli, D. (2019). Living at the extremes: Extremophiles and the limits of life in a planetary context. *Frontiers in Microbiology*, *10*, 780.

Moreno, J., López-González, J. A., Arcos-Nievas, M. A., Suárez-Estrella, F., Jurado, M. M., Estrella-González, M. J., & López, M. J. (2021). Revisiting the succession of microbial populations throughout composting: A matter of thermotolerance. *Science of the Total Environment*, *773*, 145587.

Narihiro, T., Kanosue, Y., & Hiraishi, A. (2016). Cultural, transcriptomic, and proteomic analyses of water-stressed cells of actinobacterial strains isolated from compost: Ecological implications in the fed-batch composting process. *Microbes and Environments*, ME15199.

Parikka, K. J., Jacquet, S., Colombet, J., Guillaume, D., & Le Romancer, M. (2018). Abundance and observations of thermophilic microbial and viral communities in submarine and terrestrial hot fluid systems of the French Southern and Antarctic Lands. *Polar Biology*, *41*(7), 1335–1352.

Paul, S., Choudhury, M., Deb, U., Pegu, R., Das, S., & Bhattacharya, S. S. (2019). Assessing the ecological impacts of ageing on hazard potential of solid waste landfills: A green approach through vermitechnology. *Journal of Cleaner Production*, *236*, 117643. https://doi.org/10.1016/j.jclepro.2019.117643

Piceno, Y.M., Pecora-Black, G., Kramer, S., Roy, M., Reid, F.C., Dubinsky, E.A. & Andersen, G.L., 2017. Bacterial community structure transformed after thermophilically composting human waste in Haiti. *PloS one, 12*(6), e0177626.

Rockey, N., Bischel, H. N., Kohn, T., Pecson, B., & Wigginton, K. R. (2019). The utility of flow cytometry for potable reuse. *Current Opinion in Biotechnology*, *57*, 42–49.

Ryckeboer, J., Mergaert, J., Coosemans, J., Deprins, K., & Swings, J. (2003). Microbiological aspects of biowaste during composting in a monitored compost bin. *Journal of Applied Microbiology*, *94*, 127–137.

Sarkar, S., Banerji, R., Sunanda, Chanda S., Das, P., Ganguly, S., & Pal, S. (2010). Effectiveness of inoculation with isolated *Geobacillus* strains in the thermophilic stage of vegetable waste composting. *Bioresource Technology* (Impact Factor 11.889) (97 citations), 101, 2892–2895.

Sarkar, S., Pal, S., & Chanda, S. (2016). Optimization of a vegetable waste composting process with a significant thermophilic phase. *Procedia Environmental Sciences*, *35*, 435–440.

Shin, J. H., Lee, J. W., Nam, J. H., Park, S. Y., & Lee, D. H. (2009). Bacterial community dynamics during composting of food wastes. *Korean Journal of Microbiology*, *45*(2), 148–154.

Siyambalapitiya, N., & Blackall, L. L. (2005). Discrepancies in the widely applied GAM42a fluorescence in situ hybridisation probe for Gammaproteobacteria. *FEMS Microbiology Letters*, *242*(2), 367–373.

Smaruj, P., & Bocian, K. (2020, August). Flow cytometric analysis of microorganisms. In *The book of articles national scientific conference "1st summer scientific on-line school"* (p. 87). Promovendi Foundation Publising, Poland (www.promovendi.pl).

Strom, P. F. (1985). Effect of temperature on bacterial species diversity in thermophilic solid-waste composting. *Applied and Environmental Microbiology*, *50*, 899–905.

Takaku, H., Kodaira, S., Kimoto, A., Nashimoto, M., & Takagi, M. (2006). Microbial communities in the garbage composting with rice hull as an amendment revealed by culture-dependent and culture-independent approaches. *Journal of Bioscience and Bioengineering*, *101*, 42–50.

Takebayashi, S., Narihiro, T., Fujii, Y., & Hiraishi, A. (2007). Water availability is a critical determinant of a population shift from Proteobacteria to Actinobacteria during start-up operation of mesophilic fed-batch composting. *Microbes and Environments*, *22*, 279–289.

Tang, J. C., Shibata, A., Zhou, Q., & Katayama, A. (2007). Effect of temperature on reaction rate and microbial community in composting of cattle manure with rice straw. *Journal of Bioscience and Bioengineering*, *104*, 321–328.

Vivas, A., Moreno, B., Garcia-Rodriguez, S., & Benitez, E. (2009). Assessing the impact of composting and vermicomposting on bacterial community size and structure, and microbial functional diversity of an olive-mill waste. *Bioresource Technology*, *100*, 1319–1326.

Walkley, A., & Black, I.A. (1934). An examination of the Degtjareff method for determining soil organic matter, and a proposed modification of the chromic acid titration method. *Soil Science*, *34*, 29–38.

Wideman, N. E., Oliver, J. D., Crandall, P. G., & Jarvis, N. A. (2021). Detection and potential virulence of viable but non-culturable (VBNC) Listeria monocytogenes: A review. *Microorganisms*, *9*(1), 194.

Yoon, M., Choi, J. I., & Yamashita, M. (2013). Effect of gamma irradiation on hyperthermal composting microorganisms for feasible application in space. *Advances in Space Research*, *51*(9), 1800–1807.

5 Critical Analysis of MoS_2-Based Systems for Textile Wastewater Treatment

Madhushree R, Ajay Jose, Dephan Pinheiro, and Sunaja Devi K. R.

5.1 INTRODUCTION: BASIC PROPERTIES AND IMPORTANCE OF MOS_2

As the world's environmental problems worsen, the need for sustainable and green methods to remediate them has become necessary. Excessive discharge of wastewater containing organic compounds into the environment has become a serious issue worldwide, posing a substantial risk to living beings and the ecosystem due

DOI: 10.1201/9781003499695-5

to the permanence and toxicity of these substances. Textile wastewater contains several dyes, such as methylene blue (MB), methyl orange (MO), and rhodamine B (RhB), in addition to other organic/inorganic pollutants (Wang & Mi, 2017). Inadequate treatment of textile effluents is linked to environmental degradation and a cause of various diseases, either directly or indirectly. Under light irradiation, photocatalysts can convert light energy into chemical energy and generate suitable free radicals with a redox capacity. Photocatalytic degradation of pollutants uses a photocatalyst's semiconductor features for water treatment due to its efficient light response capabilities (Li et al., 2018). On the other hand, traditional photocatalysts consisting of noble metals, such as Pt, Rh, and Ag, may have limited practical applications because of their high cost and poor abundance. Researchers have been working hard to develop novel semiconductor photocatalysts with high photo-response and practical applicability to harvest light efficiently (Mouloua et al., 2021).

In recent years, materials based on molybdenum disulfide (MoS_2), a two-dimensional (2D) layered transition metal dichalcogenide (TMDC), have attracted a lot of attention for their remarkable physical, chemical, and electrical features in the fields of optoelectronic devices and dielectric devices, such as photocatalysts, Li-ion batteries, sensors, and supercapacitors.

Bulk MoS_2 exhibits a layered structure held together by weak Van der Waals forces. A plane of Mo atoms is sandwiched between two planes of S atoms in each layer. The atoms are linked through covalent bonds. The distance between the upper and lower sulphur atoms, the crystal lattice constant, and the Mo-S length are 2.4, 3.2, and 3.1 Å, respectively (He & Que, 2016). Monolayer MoS_2 is three atoms thick and has an S-Mo-S structure (Gupta et al., 2020). Depending on the Mo atoms' coordination and stacking orientation in a single layer, there are four distinct polytypes of MoS_2: 1T, 1H, 2H, and 3R. The nature of polymorphic structures and crystal parameters are shown in Table 5.1. Trigonal prismatic coordination (D3h) of Mo atoms with distinct stacking orders is found in the 1H, 2H, and 3R polytypes, of which 1H is the most stable. This property of MoS_2 holds an advantage over graphene, allowing 2D materials to be employed in next-generation switching and optoelectronic devices (S. Wang et al., 2014). With a direct (indirect) band-gap of 1.96eV (1.2eV), MoS_2 is a semiconductor material with significant absorption in the visible region of the solar spectrum, making it suitable to be used as a co-catalyst (Jaleel et al., 2021). The detailed hexagonal structure, flower like morphology and outstanding properties of MoS_2 can be found in various literatures (Radisavljevic et al., 2011), (Chen et al., 2013), (Mouloua et al., 2021).

MoS_2-based photocatalysts, with their suitable band gaps for visible-light harvesting, have drawn considerable attention for their environmental applications, besides their other applications in areas such as hydrogen production, supercapacitors and artificial photosynthesis (Tian et al., 2020). They have low friction and, like graphite, are unaffected by oxygen and dilute acids, testifying to their robustness. The effectiveness of MoS_2 can be enhanced by doping with small amounts

TABLE 5.1 The Nature of Polymorphic Structures and Crystal Parameters of 2D MoS_2

STRUCTURE OF THE POLYMORPH	*LATTICE PARAMETERS*	*POINT GROUP*	*ELECTRONIC BEHAVIOUR*
1T	a = 5.60 Å, c = 5.99 Å	D_{6d}	Metal
2H	a = 3.15 Å, c = 12.30 Å	D_{6h}	Semiconductor
3R	a = 3.17 Å, c = 18.38 Å	C_{3v}	semiconductor

of other noble metals. Because of their high UV/visible-light absorption capacity, oxidation potential, chemical stability, low toxicity, outstanding charge-storage ability, and cycling performance, nanostructured metals have been widely exploited as promising photocatalysts for the mineralization of organic contaminants (Voiry et al., 2015). MoS_2 also has a high adsorption capacity and an adjustable band structure. Due to these mentioned advantages, MoS_2 has been widely employed as a co-photocatalyst in the manufacture of composites, particularly in the photocatalytic removal of organic pollutants. MoS_2-based materials have significantly developed in hydrogen evolution reaction (HER), energy conversion, and storage. MoS_2 with an odd number of layers has the potential to produce oscillating piezoelectric voltage and current outputs, implying that it might be utilized to power nanodevices and stretchable electronics (Li & Zhu, 2015; Taiwo et al., 2020).

Herein, we summarize work in the preparation methods, properties, and applications of MoS_2-based catalysts in photocatalytic dye degradation. The recent developments in modifying the properties of MoS_2 upon doping with one or two other components leading to binary and ternary systems based on MoS_2 (MoS_2 as a co-catalyst) are also discussed.

5.2 GENERAL METHODS EMPLOYED FOR THE PREPARATION OF MOS_2 AND MOS_2-BASED SYSTEMS

Several studies have been reported on the different methods for preparing MoS_2. Chemical vapor deposition (He & Que, 2016; Mouloua et al., 2021; Wang et al., 2013), hydrothermal processes (Cao et al., 2017; Chaudhary et al., 2018; He & Que, 2016; Muralikrishna et al., 2015; Nagaraju et al., 2007; Tao et al., 2014; W. Wang et al., 2014; Ye et al., 2014; X. H. Zhang et al., 2016; Zhou et al., 2011), solvo-thermal processes (Vattikuti et al., 2015; R. Z. Zhang et al.,

2019), hydrothermal exfoliation (Liu et al., 2014; Zhang et al., 2015) electrochemical exfoliation (Qin et al., 2016; Tao et al., 2014), chemical exfoliation (Duphil & Le, 2002; Li & Zhu, 2015; J. Liu et al., 2012), MoS_2 sulphurization (Lin et al., 2012), liquid-assisted grinding (Tang et al., 2020), hydrothermal inter-calcination exfoliation (Liu et al., 2013; Zhao et al., 2015a), and microwave-assisted methods (Panigrahi & Pathak, 2011; Tang et al., 2017; Xue et al., 2018) are among the most significant.

Top-down processes like mechanical exfoliation and chemical exfoliation, and bottom-up processes, such as chemical vapour deposition (CVD), physical vapour transport, and wet chemical methods, can synthesize two-dimensional MoS_2. The mechanical cleavage approach was used to create monolayer MoS_2 for the first time (He & Que, 2016). All the different synthetic processes have their advantages and drawbacks. Chemical exfoliation, in contrast to mechanical exfoliation, is capable of creating vast amounts of mono- or few-layered MoS_2 nanosheets with relatively good carrier mobility (Han et al., 2021).

5.2.1 Hydrothermal Approach

By modifying the hydrothermal reaction time and temperature, MoS_2 nanosheets with a highly crystalline nature and different morphology can be fabricated (Liu et al., 2012). Li et al. previously observed that synthesis at low temperatures $(130-150°C)$ produces amorphous MoS_2 nanospheres with no evidence of layered material (Vattikuti et al., 2015). Temperature and time length, on the other hand, significantly impact morphology and crystalline size. Nagaraju et al. reported on the hydrothermal synthesis of MoS_2 nanosheets at 180°C, where they observed poor MoS_2 crystals (2007). The procedure followed for synthesizing MoS_2 nanosheets via the hydrothermal method is as follows: 3 mmol sodium molybdate and 9 mmol thioacetamide were completely dissolved in 50 mL distilled water. 2.8 mmol of sillicontungstic acid was added to this colourless solution, stirring continuously. The 50-ml reaction solution was tightly sealed and held at a temperature of 220°C for 24 h in a 100-ml stainless Teflon-lined autoclave. The black precipitate was filtered and washed several times with NaOH solution, ethanol, and distilled water before vacuum drying at 60°C for 5 h (Chaudhary et al., 2018). A similar protocol has been followed for the synthesis of bilayer MoS_2 nanosheets (Cao et al., 2017; Muralikrishna et al., 2015; Nagaraju et al., 2007; Ye et al., 2014; X. H. Zhang et al., 2016).

5.2.2 Exfoliation Process

The exfoliation method includes chemical exfoliation (Duphil & Le, 2002; Li & Zhu, 2015; J. Liu et al., 2012) and electrochemical exfoliation, where a positive bias is applied to the working electrode during the process (Qin et al., 2016; Tao et al., 2014). In addition, 1T metallic MoS_2 can be established through the ion intercalation process, hydrothermal inter-calcination exfoliation (Liu et al., 2013; Zhao et al., 2015), and hydrothermal exfoliation (Liu et al., 2014; Zhang et al., 2015). Exfoliation helps to synthesize both monolayer and few-layer MoS_2 nanosheets (Wang & Mi, 2017). Sonication can effectively disperse MoS_2 in a solution via liquid-phase exfoliation, a form of ultrasonic exfoliation. This method preserves the semiconductor properties of MoS_2 nanosheets compared to lithium-ion intercalation. The exfoliation method is straightforward, rapid, and scalable, and it may also be used to prepare other transition metal dichalcogenides.

5.2.3 Chemical Vapour Deposition

Chemical vapour deposition has frequently been employed to make high-quality atomic thin MoS_2. MoS_2 is synthesized via CVD to sulphurize MoO_3 (Lin et al., 2012). CVD technologies, such as SiO_2/Si, sapphire, polyimide, and others, could be used to generate large-area SiO_2 flakes on substrates (He & Que, 2016; Mouloua et al., 2021; Wang et al., 2013). The growth temperature of MoS_2 can be reduced to $150-300°C$ using plasma-enhanced chemical vapour deposition (PECVD), making it possible to deposit MoS_2 directly on plastic substrates (Ahn et al., 2015).

5.3 CHARACTERIZATION OF MOS_2

The X-ray diffraction (XRD) patterns of MoS_2 show four peaks at 14.2, 33.4, 39.8, and 58.8° corresponding to the hexagonal MoS_2 (002), (100), (103), and (110) reflection planes (X. H. Zhang et al., 2016). But the two most evident diffraction peaks occur at 27.4° and 13.1° $(\text{JCPDS } 37-1492)$, which are due to the (002) and (100) planes, respectively (Babu Christus et al., 2019; Nagaraju et al., 2007; Zhou et al., 2011). The sharp and high diffraction peak indexed at (002) indicates the formation of a well-stacked layered MoS_2 structure during the hydrothermal process. The different planes corresponding to MoS_2 and other doped metals/metal oxides/composites will be observed in the XRD of binary or ternary composites, indicating that MoS_2 does not disturb the lattice of the composite structure (Qin et al., 2016; Tao et al., 2014; Vattikuti & Byon, 2017). The XRD pattern of the MoS_2 is shown in Figure 5.1(a).

In the Fourier Transform Infrared Spectroscopy (FTIR) spectra of MoS_2, it is observed that the band at 667 cm^{-1} corresponds to Mo-S bonding, the band at 802 cm^{-1} is due to the S–S bond, and those at 1399 and 1626 cm^{-1} are because of hydroxyl group stretching vibrations and Mo–O vibrations, as depicted in

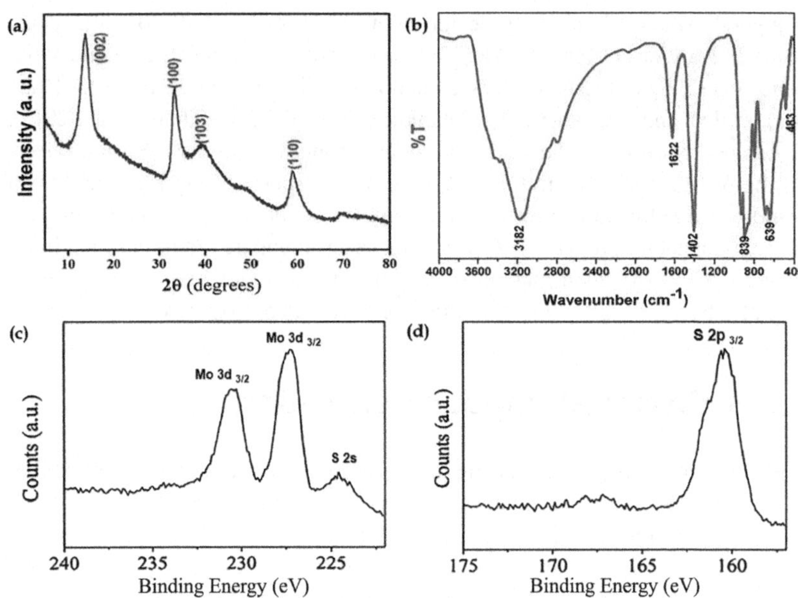

FIGURE 5.1 (a) XRD pattern, (b) FTIR spectrum, (c) XPS Mo 3D spectrum, and (d) XPS S 2p spectrum of MoS_2. Reprinted with the permission of (a) Royal Society of Chemistry from (Muralikrishna et al., 2015). (b) Elsevier (X. Zhang et al., 2019). (c) and (d) Elsevier from (Yang et al., 2017).

Figure 5.1(b) (Nagaraju et al., 2007; Zhang et al., 2019). The X-ray photoelectron spectroscopy (XPS) spectrum investigates the chemical states, surface chemical composition, and oxidation states. The deconvoluted XPS spectra of the hybrid composite consist of Mo-3D core level peaks of commercial MoS_2 nanosheets (231.6, 228.9, 228, 226 eV). The binding energy corresponding to 231.6 eV and 228.9 eV has $3d_{5/2}$ and $3d_{3/2}$ bands with Mo^{6+} and Mo^{4+} states, respectively (Gopika et al., 2019). XPS of MoS_2 The Mo 3D spectrum and S 2p spectrum with high resolution are depicted in Figures 5.1(c) and 5.1(d).

Scanning electron microscopy (SEM) measurements were used to examine the size and morphologies of the synthesized MoS_2. Li et al. studied the morphology of the synthesized MoS_2, which resulted in flower- and tube-like nanostructures, as shown in Figure 5.2(a,b) (2004). Nanosheets synthesized via chemical exfoliation resulted in a sheet-like morphology (Lukowski et al., 2013), as shown in Figure 5.2(c). The samples comprise several aggregated nanosheets, as illustrated in Figure 5.2(d). High-magnification morphology studies using SEM images demonstrate that the collected samples are primarily made up of well-defined nanosheets with lateral sizes ranging from 200 to 400 nm. The product yield with the foil-like thin sheet morphology was nearly 100% (Zhang et al.,

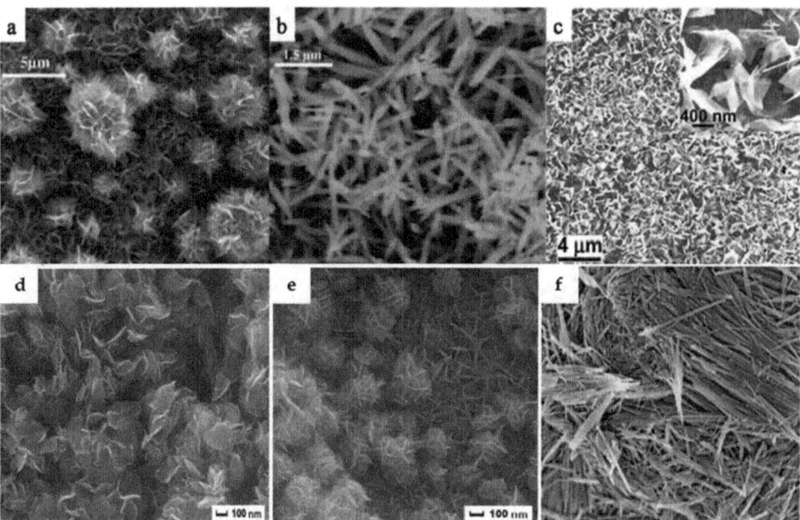

FIGURE 5.2 SEM images of MoS_2: (a) nanoflower, (b) nanotubes, (c)–(d) nanosheets, (e) nanosphere, and (f) nanofiber. Reprinted with permission of (a,b) Wiley and (c) ACS publications from (Li et al., 2004; Lukowski et al., 2013), (d) Chalcogenide Letters from (X. H. Zhang et al., 2016), (e) Elsevier from (Xu et al., 2014), (f) Springer from (Nagaraju et al., 2007)

2016). Figure 5.2(e) illustrates that the flower-like nanospheres are composed of MoS_2 nanosheets and that their sizes range between 50 and 100 nm (Xu et al., 2014). SEM images reveal MoS_2 nanofibers with a diameter of 120–300 nm (Figure 5.2(f)), which are perfectly aligned and appear as a cluster of bundles, as the nanofibers are self-assembled into bundles (Nagaraju et al., 2007).

5.4 MODIFIED MOS_2 SYSTEMS

MoS_2, as a unique representative of layered materials, has been extensively investigated as a co-catalyst for the photodegradation of pollutants. It can be used with several materials such as graphene, carbon nitride, and TiO_2 to improve photocatalytic degradation where the composites have shown an improvement in properties compared to pure MoS_2. Fabricating MoS_2 with other comparable metals/metal ions or semiconducting materials results in the formation of binary and tertiary composites/systems, collectively called modified MoS_2 systems (Cao et al., 2021).

Of all the methods mentioned, the formation of heterostructures can significantly improve photocatalytic properties by effectively separating photogenerated electron-hole pairs (McDaniel et al., 2011). Charge carriers can migrate across the heterostructure's interface, thus inhibiting the recombination rate. Binary and ternary combinations play a key role in pollution reduction and environmental-energy storage device applications through photocatalytic technology (Wang et al., 2017; Hasija et al., 2019).

5.4.1 Binary Systems

Binary systems involving MoS_2 are prepared using various methods such as hydrothermal, CVD, solvothermal, and exfoliation methods. First, after MoS_2 is prepared using a suitable method mentioned earlier, it is dissolved in a solvent, followed by exfoliation via ultrasonication. The secondary material is then added to this, stirred well, centrifuged, washed, and dried overnight at 100° C. The composite is then calcined at the designated 5–6 h temperature. Several binary systems of MoS_2 with single metals or semiconducting materials such as Ti, TiO_2 (Cao et al., 2021; Chandrabose et al., 2021), and NiS_2 (Harish et al., 2021) have been prepared.

5.4.2 Ternary Systems

The preparation of ternary systems follows a protocol similar to that for binary systems, where a third material is added along with the secondary material to the $g-C_3N_4$. The major ternary systems prepared and studied include MoS_2 /TiO_2 /$g-C_3N_4$ (Jaleel et al., 2021), Bi_2S_3/MoS_2/TiO_2 (Drmosh et al., 2020), MoS_2/Al_2O_3/$g-C_3N_4$ (Vattikuti & Byon, 2017), and Co - g - C_3N_4/MoS_2 (Chen et al., 2019) are discussed in the next section. A summary of the photocatalytic degradation of modified MoS_2-binary (Table 5.2) and ternary (Table 5.3) composites with their applications in various dye degradations is explained in a later section.

5.5 MODIFIED MOS_2 SYSTEMS FOR WASTEWATER TREATMENT

Dye residues are present in substantial quantities in textile industry effluents, and these are the principal contaminants harming water bodies. Approximately $20-30\%$ of the dyestuff used in the dyeing process is discharged into water

TABLE 5.2 Summary of Photocatalytic Degradation of Modified MoS_2-Binary Composites

CATALYST	*LIGHT SOURCE*	*CONTAMINANT*	*INITIAL CONCENTRATION*	*PHOTOCATALYTIC EFFICIENCY (%)/ REACTION TIME (MIN)*	*REF*
MoS_2	Natural light	CV	5 mg/50 mL	92/50	(Sharma et al., 2021)
MoS_2	300-W incandescent lamp	CR	10 mg/80 mL	75/80	(Ullah et al., 2021)
MoS_2/TiO_2	320, 300-W lamp	MB	25 mg/50 mL	100/60	(Chandrabose et al., 2021)
GO/MoS_2	Hg lamp	MB	50 mL 15 mg/L	100/50	(Yuan et al., 2017)
$SrFe_{12}O_{19}/MoS_2$	Natural light	MB	20 mg/L	97/-	(Chen et al., 2021)
rGO/MoS_2	SOL2/500S lamp	MB	8.5 mL 12.5 mg/L	96/300	(Cravanzola et al., 2016)
TiO_2 NTs/MoS_2	500-W Xe lamp	RhB MB	20 mg/L	76 100	(Cao et al., 2021)
Ag_3PO_4/MoS_2	350-W Xe lamp	MB RhB MO Phenol	30 mL 20 mg/L 30 mL 20 mg/L 30 mL 10 mg/L 30 mL 5 mg/L	98/60 100/80 100/120 95/200	(Zhu et al., 2016)
$ZnO/MoS_2/rGO$	Natural light source	MB Carbendazim	50 mL 15.9 mg/L	98/60 97/60	(Kumar et al., 2016)
$MoS_2/g\text{-}C_3N_4$	500-W Xe lamp	MO	50 mL 20 mg/L	60/300	(Peng & Li, 2014)

(Continued)

TABLE 5.2 (Continued)

CATALYST	*LIGHT SOURCE*	*CONTAMINANT*	*INITIAL CONCENTRATION*	*PHOTOCATALYTIC EFFICIENCY (%)/ REACTION TIME (MIN)*	*REF*
MoS_2/NiS_2	Xe lamp	RhB	2 mg/100 mL	90.5/32	(Harish et al., 2021)
MoS_2/g-C_3N_4	250-W metal halide lamp	MO CIP TC	10 mL 10 mg/L	92.4/120 81/240 96/240	(Lu et al., 2016)
TiO_2/MoS_2	300-W Xe lamp	phenol	60 mL 10 mg/L	78% (in 150 min)	(Wang et al., 2016)
Ag-doped MoS_2	Using reducing agent ($NaBH_4$)	MB (10 ppm)	4 mg/10 mL	100	(Ikram et al., 2020)
SnO_2-MoS_2 nanostructures (NSs)	Visible light	MB MR (100 ppm)	0.5 mg	58.5/120 and 94/120	(Rani et al., 2019)
MoS_2/Bi_2O_3	150-W Xe lamp	Crystal Violet (CV)	25 mg/50 mL	100 Complete degradation	(Goud et al., 2020)
MoS_2/BiOBr	300-W Xe lamp	RhB	100 mL 10 mg/L	94/50	(Di et al., 2014)
MoS_2/Wurtzite ZnS	Xe lamp	CV	10 mg	98.5/40	(Rao Akshatha et al., 2020)
MoS_2 nanoflakes photoanode on Ti foil	300-W Xe arc lamp	RhB 4-CP	1 mg/L	90/-	(Zhou et al., 2019)
MoS_2/NiFe LDH	Solar light	RhB 20 ppm	20 mg/20 mL	90/120	(Nayak et al., 2019)

Co-doped MoS_2	visible light	MB 5 ppm	10 mg	96/90	(Raza et al., 2020)
(MNPs) MoS_2@Au hybrid	300-W Xe lamp	RhB 20 ppm	20 mg//L	90/40	(Lai et al., 2019)
g-C_3N_4/MoS_2	Ultrasonic bath	Levofloxacin MB 10 ppm	10 mg/L	75.81/140 98.43/14	(He et al., 2020)
Nickel (Ni)-doped MoS_2	500-W Hg lamp as resource UV light	MB and RhB 30 ppm	10 mg/30 mL	96/90 and 91/90	(Khan et al., 2020)
MoS_2 NFs/TiO_2 (B)	250-W lamp	RhB 30 ppm	20 mg/100 mL	80/60	(Paul et al., 2018)
MoS_2/YVO_4 Composite	350-W Xe lamp	MO 20 ppm	25 mg	60/-	(Chen et al., 2018)
MoS_2 QDs/g-C_3N_4	350-W Xe lamp	RhB 10 ppm	25 mg/50 mL	99/9	(Fu et al., 2017)
Bi_2S_3/MoS_2	35-W Xe lamp	PR 100 ppm	5 mg/50 mL	83.4/90	(Vattikuti & Byon, 2016)
MoS_2 nanoflower	Natural sunlight	MB CV 30 ppm	20 mg/100 mL	99.3/40	(Sadhanala et al., 2018)
Montmorillonite@MoS_2/CdS composite	300-W xenon lamp	RhB 100 ppm	10 mg/100 mL	98.9/45	(Peng et al., 2019)
MoS_2 nanosheets loaded ZnO–g-C_3N_4	Visible-light irradiation	MB atrazine	15 mg	99.5/30 84.9/30	(Jo et al., 2016)

TABLE 5.3 Summary of Photocatalytic Degradation of Modified MoS_2-Ternary Composites

CATALYST	*LIGHT SOURCE*	*CONTAMINANTS*	*INITIAL CONCENTRATION*	*PHOTOCATALYTIC EFFICIENCY % REACTION TIME (MIN)*	*REF*
$MoS_2/g\text{-}C_3N_4/TiO_2$	75-W halogen lamp	MG (10 ppm)	50 mg	86/60	(Jaleel et al., 2021)
$Bi_2S_3/MoS_2/TiO_2$	250-W Xenon	MB 10 ppm	10 mg/200 mL	99/40	(Drmosh et al., 2020)
$MoS_2/Al_2O_3/g\text{-}C_3N_4$	150-W tungsten halogen lamp	CV (100 ppm)	5 mg/100 mL	97/90	(Vattikuti & Byon, 2017)
RGO-MoS_2-$NiCo_2O_4$	Visible light irradiation	RhB (10 ppm)	50 mg	95/90	(Chakrabarty et al., 2018)
Fe_3O_4@MoS_2/Ag_3PO_4	500-W Xe lamp	RhB CR	0.2 mg/mL	98.9/10 and 90.74/10	(Guo et al., 2016)
Co-$g\text{-}C_3N_4/MoS_2$	300-W Xe lamp	RhB	20 mg/L	94/150	(Chen et al., 2019)
$g\text{-}C_3N_4/Ag/MoS_2$	300-W Xenon arc lamp	RhB (20 ppm)	100 mg/100 mL	66.47/60	(Dingze et al., 2016)
$TiO_2/g\text{-}C_3N_4/MoS_2$	XG500 xenon long-arc lamp.	MO	20 mg/L	90.04/60	(W. Zhang et al., 2016)
MoS_2 incorporated $\alpha\text{-}Fe_2O_3/ZnO$	500-W mercury-xenon lamp	RhB (10 ppm) ciprofloxacin (50 ppm)	50 mg	91/- 83/-	(Tama et al., 2019)

bodies as effluents (Duphil & Le, 2002). The dyes that are released can be extremely harmful, with several of these being carcinogenic, contaminating both ground and surface water. As a result, effective strategies for removing organic contaminants from effluents must be established (Theerthagiri et al., 2017).

The degradation of harmful organic pollutants has been used as a model to assess the photocatalytic efficacy of various samples, binary systems, and ternary systems, including MoS_2. Various dyes have been studied using MoS_2- based catalysts, among which few are discussed in this section. Jaleel et al. studied the degradation of 10 ppm MG using 50 mg of MoS_2/ g-C_3N_4/TiO_2 under visible light, resulting in 97% degradation efficiency in 60 min (Jaleel et al., 2021). Chandrabose et al. studied the degradation of 10–50 ppm MB using 25 mg of MoS_2/TiO_2 under Asahi Spectra HAL 320, 300 W, obtaining 100% removal efficiency within 1 h (2021). Degradation of MB was studied using 15 mg of MoS_2/GO under a mercury lamp, resulting in complete degradation under 50 min (Yuan et al., 2017). Chen et al. achieved 97% degradation efficiency for MB dye using 20 mg $SrFe_{12}O_{19}$/ MoS_2 under a natural light source (2021). A reduced-GO/MoS_2 was studied for degradation of MB dye by Cravanzola et al. using 12.5 mg of catalyst under a SOL2/500Wlamp, resulting in 96% degradation efficiency in 5 h (2016). Cao et al. prepared Ti-modified MoS_2 nanotubes for the degradation of MB using a 500-W Xe lamp and obtained degradation efficiency of about 76% (2021). Using 10 mg of Bi_2S_3/MoS_2/TiO_2 and 10 ppm of MB, degradation was studied under a 250-W Xenon lamp, showed outstanding degradation efficiency of 99% in just 4 min (Drmosh et al., 2020). Zhu et al. studied the degradation of MB using 20 mg Ag_3PO_4/MoS_2 under a 350-W Xe lamp, resulting in 98% degradation efficiency in 60 min (2016). Kumar et al. studied the degradation of MB using 15.9 mg of ZnO/MoS_2/RGO under natural light, showed 98% removal capacity in 60 min (2016). Ag-doped MoS_2, under the influence of a reducing agent ($NaBH_4$), resulted in complete degradation of 10ppm MB dye (Ikram et al., 2020). Rani et al. used 0.5 mg of SnO_2 - MoS_2 under visible light, for photocatalytic degradation of MB and MR dyes which resulted in 58.5 and 94% removal efficiency in 120 min (2019). Raza et al., achieved 96% degradation for 5ppm MG dye using Co doped MoS_2 (Raza et al., 2020).

Cao et al. prepared TiO_2/MoS_2 nanotubes for the degradation of RhB using a 500-W Xe lamp achieved complete degradation (2021). Using 20 mg Ag_3PO_4/MoS_2, Zhu et al. studied the degradation of RhB under a 350-W Xe lamp, resulted in 100% degradation efficiency in 80 min (2016). Harish et al. reported 90% degradation in 32 min for RhB dye using MoS_2/NiS_2 (2021). MoS_2/BiOBr was used to study RhB under a 300W Xe lamp, resulting in removal capacity in 50 min (Di et al., 2014). MoS_2/NiFe LDH composite showed 90% degradation efficiency in 120 min for RhB dye (Nayak et al., 2019). Ni- doped MoS_2 showed up to 96% and 90% photocatalytic degradation efficiency in 90 and 40 min, for MB and RhB dyes for respectively (Khan et al., 2020; Lai et al., 2019). Montmorillonite/CdS modification on MoS_2 showed 98% removal capacity in 45 min towards 100ppm RhB dye (Peng et al., 2019).

Peng and Li studied the degradation of Methyl orange MO using 20 mg of $MoS_2/g-C_3N_4$ under a 500-W Xe lamp and found 60% degradation efficiency in 5 h (2014). Using 10 mg Ag_3PO_4/MoS_2, Zhu et al. studied the degradation of MO under a 350-W Xe lamp, resulted in complete removal of dye in 120 min (2016). Lu et al. studied the degradation of MO using 10 mg of $MoS_2/g-C_3N_4$ under a metal halide lamp, which resulted in 92% in 2 h (2016). Further, MoS_2/YVO_4 catalyst showed 60% degradation efficiency for 20 ppm MO dye (Chen et al., 2018).

Goud et al. studied the degradation of crystal violet (CV) using 25 mg of MoS_2/Bi_2O_3 under a 150-W Xe lamp and found complete degradation (2020). Rao Akshatha et al. synthesized MoS_2/Wurtzite ZnS and studied the degradation of CV under a Xe lamp, which resulted in 98% degradation in 40 min (2020). 99% degradation efficiency was obtained using MoS_2 nanoflakes for removal of CV dye (Sadhanala et al., 2018). Rani et al. used 0.5 mg of SnO_2-MoS_2 for the degradation of methylene red (MR) under visible light, resulting in 90% degradation efficiency in 120 min (2019).

Zhu et al. studied degradation of phenol using 5 mg Ag_3PO_4/MoS_2 under a 350-W Xe lamp, with degradation efficiency of 95% in 200 min (2016). TiO_2/MoS_2 was also studied under a 300-W Xe lamp and resulted in 78% dye removal efficiency in 150 min (Wang et al., 2016). Kumar et al. studied degradation of Carbendazim using 15 mg of ZnO/MoS_2/RGO under natural light, with 97% efficiency in 60 min (2016). A well-known modified MoS_2 binary system is $MoS_2/g-C_3N_4$ was studied by Lu et al. for the degradation of Ciprofloxacin (CIP) and tetracycline (TC) under a 250-W metal halide lamp, resulted in 81% and 96% degradation efficiency in 4 h (2016). Other toxic organic/inorganic dyes were also studied. Zhou et al., worked on 4-chlorophenol using Ti/MoS_2 under a 300-W Xe lamp, and resulted in removal efficiency of 85% (2019). Under similar experimental conditions, other common dyes such as Levofloxacin (Yanhhing He et al., 2020), atrazine (Wan-Kuen Jo et al., 2016), and phenol red (Vattikuti & Byon, 2016) were studied.

From the literature, high degradation efficiency can be achieved in the presence of light and with the use of a catalyst over a set period of time. To reach adsorption-desorption equilibrium, a suspension was placed in the dark for 15 min in a standard reaction technique. A UV-vis spectrophotometer was used to measure the concentration of the solution at regular intervals. Time, light intensity, dye concentration, catalyst quantity, pH conditions, and other variables were tuned to achieve maximum dye degradation.

The catalyst's reusability is a critical factor in determining its utility in practical and industrial applications. A catalyst's reusability indicates its resilience and, as a result, its utility. Many researchers have concentrated their efforts on developing a catalyst that can operate for a longer period of time. Most of the time, after a few cycles, a minor decrease in photocatalytic activity of the nanocomposite is seen, which could be attributed to dye molecules occupying active sites of the nanocomposite during the reusability process.

5.6 MECHANISM OF DEGRADATION OF TEXTILE DYES

Based on the band theory of semiconductors, photocatalysis involves the following steps: (1) photon absorption; (2) charge separation (electron-hole pair formation) within the photocatalyst; and (3) subsequent production of reactive oxygen species (ROS), which are responsible for the activity or advanced oxidation process. In order to elucidate the complete mechanism of photocatalytic dye degradation by MoS_2-based systems, we need to investigate each of these steps individually.

5.6.1 Excitation: Photon Absorption

The primary requirement for a photocatalytic process is a suitable light source. All photocatalytic processes are initiated by the absorption of photon, which can lead to electron excitation from the ground state. The excitation process depends on the band gap of the material as well as the intensity of the incoming photons. Hence a photocatalytic process cannot be activated by any source of light.

5.6.2 Separation: Electron–Hole Pair Formation

MoS_2 is commonly used as a co-catalyst in most photocatalytic reactions. Generally, MoS_2 is introduced into a photocatalytic system to support or enhance its innate ability. Hence, there are binary and tertiary hybrid photocatalytic systems with varying concentrations of MoS_2. In order to elucidate the proper mechanism of photocatalytic activity, we need to assess the nature of materials in the hybrid system. Based on the type of heterojunction formed, we can determine how electron–hole formation and charge separation take place, leading to the formation of the observed ROS. Excitation of electrons and formation of charge carriers are the key steps in the whole process, which are discussed subsequently.

5.6.3 Dye Degradation: Advanced Oxidation Process

The different types of ROS produced during a photocatalytic process are superoxide anion radical, hydrogen peroxide, hydroxyl radical, and singlet oxygen. Although these can be formed directly from the substrates (water and oxygen) from the redox potential of the charge carriers, as explained above, the possibility of secondary ROS formed from initially formed or primary ROS cannot be neglected. Sometimes we observe that one or more of the ROS responsible for dye degradation may not be the primary ROS. In such cases, the best explanation will be the formation of a secondary ROS, which is more stable in the liquid medium. This parallel formation of ROS depends mainly on the pH of the solution and solvent and is often a missed detail while explaining the mechanism.

Hence a photocatalytic scheme is best explained based on the direct and parallel formation of ROS. Among the listed ROS, OH radicals can be formed directly (when the valence band potential of the holes is high) as well as parallelly. One experimental method is to add hole scavengers to prove the existence of OH radicals from VB and secondary OH radicals. However, superoxide anion radical is a common primary ROS. Hydrogen peroxide and singlet oxygen are believed to be secondary ROS in most cases since both conduction band (CB) and valence band (VB) potentials do not have any effect in the formation of the same. One should note that the charge carriers or holes and electrons can also participate directly in dye degradation without the need for ROS production.

5.6.4 Photocatalytic Schemes Based on Types of Heterojunctions

(a) Conventional Photocatalysis with Pure MoS_2

In most published works, MoS_2 is reported as a co-catalyst rather than a pure photocatalytic material. Hence, many photocatalytic hybrid systems containing MoS_2 are reported every day. The advantages of these hybrid systems are primarily efficient charge separation and their subsequent migration, which retards the rate of recombination, which enhances the whole photocatalytic reaction (Zhang, et al., 2021). Hence, the development of composites with MoS_2 or heterojunctions of MoS_2 with a known photocatalyst such as metals, non-metals, polymers, or other semiconductors is an easy way to solve the recombination problem. However, in the case of photocatalytic systems with more than one phase (different crystal structures of the same material) or material (MoS_2-based photocatalytic systems), it is necessary to understand the underlying mechanism of charge migration and separation. Depending on the pathway of charge migration, which depends on the position of CB and VB of the ingredient materials in the system, the following concepts or photocatalytic schemes for binary systems are developed.

(b) Type II Heterojunction Photocatalysis

This is the most-reported traditional photocatalytic scheme for hybrid photocatalytic systems. Two semiconductor materials with different band positions form an interface, which can result in band alignment and a new path for electron migration. Based on the conduction band positions of the component materials, three types of conventional heterojunctions are possible (Huang et al., 2019; Low et al., 2017).

Among the three types, the most feasible and reported heterojunctions are type II heterojunction photocatalyst systems, where electron migration seems to be more favourable than the others (Low et al., 2017). For the formation of a type II heterojunction, the materials forming the interface must have a higher CB and VB than the other. Even though this promotes efficient charge separation, the resultant potential of the charge carrier is reduced in such a way that inhibits photocatalysis. For type II heterojunctions, it is not necessary that both the interfacial materials be semiconductors (Low et al., 2017).

(c) p-n Junction Scheme Photocatalysis

A p-n junction scheme can be viewed as a modified or revised version of type II heterojunction scheme. A heterojunction formed from interfacing one n-type and a p-type semiconductor is termed a p-n junction photocatalytic system (Low et al., 2017). The difference between p-n junction and type II heterojunction is that the former forms an internal electric field prior to illumination, while the later needs illumination for charge migration and electric field formation (Xu et al., 2018). Several MoS_2 composites form p-n junction systems, as MoS_2 behaves as a p-type semiconductor (Xu et al., 2018). A typical p-n junction photocatalytic scheme for a MoS_2-based system is the MoS_2–CdS interface (Y. Liu et al., 2013).

(d) Z-Scheme Photocatalysis

The photocatalytic scheme that follows type II heterojunction and p-n junction schemes is called Z-scheme (Zhang et al., 2020). Based on the direction of electric field, this pathway of charge carriers resemble the letter z, hence the name Z-scheme (Xu et al., 2018). In both p-n junction and Z-scheme pathways, we assume the formation of an internal electric field. The semiconductor properties of the materials involved result in the internal electric field, charge distribution, and band edge bending, which ultimately decide the fate of the charge transfer pathway upon illumination (Xu et al., 2018).

A Bi_2WO_6 composite with MoS_2 is an example of a direct z-scheme (Liang et al., 2021). While a dual z-scheme mechanism is observed for MoS_2/g-C_3N_4/TiO_2 heterostructure, a ternary composite (Jaleel & Devi, 2020). Moreover, MoS_2-based ternary catalysts undergo photocatalytic all-solid-state z-scheme, or indirect z-scheme (Wang et al., 2020; Zeng et al., 2019).

(e) Dual Z-Scheme Photocatalysis

For ternary photocatalytic systems with MoS_2, a dual Z-scheme pathway is also possible. Drmosh et al. (2020) prepared a ternary composite Bi_2S_3/MoS_2/TiO_2 under UV-vis irradiation. There are two alternative charge transfer channels that can be explored based on the respective energy band levels of Bi_2S_3, MoS_2, and TiO_2 to explain the improvement in photocatalytic performance: type II and Z-scheme heterojunctions.

In the case of type II heterojunction, the e^-/h^+ pairs generated by photons are successfully separated; however, it results in a lower redox ability. The electrons from the CB of Bi_2S_3 and MoS_2 will move towards TiO_2's CB, and the holes from the VB of TiO_2 will be transferred to the VB of Bi_2S_3. Considering Z-scheme heterojunction, the photogenerated electrons in TiO_2's CB will recombine with the generated holes in MoS_2's VB (first Z-scheme pathway), and the electrons in the CB of MoS_2 recombine with the VB holes of Bi_2S_3 (second Z-scheme pathway). This double/dual Z-scheme mechanism results in the availability of electrons in the CB of Bi_2S_3, which has a high reduction potential, and therefore quickly reduces O_2 and holes in the VB of TiO_2 and is capable of oxidizing water and generating hydroxyl radicals, which can either degrade the organic contaminants or undergo additional oxidation.

(f) S-Scheme Photocatalysis

A huge disadvantage in electron migration based on type II heterojunction is that the chances of like charge repulsions are high (Xu et al., 2020). Recently a scheme called S-scheme has been proposed (Xu et al., 2020). One could argue that this is a revised version of Z-scheme photocatalysis in which the combining materials are identified as either reduction photocatalysts or oxidation photocatalysts based on their band positions (Zhang et al., 2019; Xu et al., 2020).

Based on the Fermi levels, MoS_2 is an oxidative photocatalyst (lower Fermi level, 0.24 V), and $CdIn_2S_4$ is a reduction-type photocatalyst (higher Fermi level, −0.221 V). An internal electric field is generated when two different Fermi levels of semiconductors come in contact. The electrons flow into the system until they remain constant from a lower Fermi level $\left(CdIn_2S_4\right)$ to higher Fermi level $\left(MoS_2\right)$. $CdIn_2S_4$ and MoS_2 are negatively and positively charged, respectively. At the interface, an internal electric field is successfully formed. Barrier zones created in $CdIn_2S_4$ are due to the loss of electrons (band edge bends upside), and no movement of electrons from this site to MoS_2 takes place. Similarly, the movement of holes is hindered (band edge bends downside), and no holes transfer from this site to $CdIn_2S_4$. Under the irradiation of sunlight, the photo-induced electron/hole pair is generated. The electrons in the CB of MoS_2 and holes in the VB of $CdIn_2S_4$ will recombine due to the internal electric field generated as a result of the synergic effect. But the holes in the VB of MoS_2 and electrons in the CB of $CdIn_2S_4$ will remain motionless. This S-scheme mechanism would result in excellent photocatalytic activity.

5.7 CONCLUSION

In this chapter, we have discussed the recent progress made in the synthesis of MoS_2 and MoS_2-based composite systems. MoS_2 nanomaterials are excellent materials for designing composites for the photocatalytic degradation of pollutants present in wastewater. Properties like ease of synthesis, several available methods of preparation, low toxicity, stability, appropriate band gap, absorption capability assisted by its large surface area, and reusability make MoS_2 an outstanding candidate as a photocatalyst. The structural and morphological aspects of MoS_2 are also discussed. However, MoS_2 does have some downsides. One way of improving the properties of MoS_2 is by adding other materials, notably metals and metal ions, to fabricate binary and ternary systems of MoS_2. Such composites have significantly better properties suited for photocatalytic applications and have been extensively used in dye degradation and water treatment applications. Further, the plausible and exact mechanism of the photodegradation in many of the MoS_2 and MoS_2-based composites were briefly discussed. It is hoped that this chapter will help in the exploration of novel, non-toxic, light-stable, scalable, and inexpensive MoS_2-based catalysts for various applications.

ACKNOWLEDGEMENTS

The authors are grateful to express their gratitude to Christ (Deemed to be University), Bangalore, for their support and encouragement.

REFERENCES

Ahn, C., Lee, J., Kim, H. U., Bark, H., Jeon, M., Ryu, G. H., Lee, Z., Yeom, G. Y., Kim, K., Jung, J., Kim, Y., Lee, C., & Kim, T. (2015). Low-temperature synthesis of large-scale molybdenum disulfide thin films directly on a plastic substrate using plasma-enhanced chemical vapor deposition. *Advanced Materials*, 27, 5223–5229. https://doi.org/10.1002/adma.201501678

Babu Christus, A. A., Panneerselvam, P., Ravikumar, A., Marieeswaran, M., & Sivanesan, S. (2019). MoS_2 nanosheet mediated ZnO-g-C3N 4 nanocomposite as a peroxidase mimic: Catalytic activity and application in the colorimetric determination of Hg(ii). *RSC Advances*, *9*, 4268–4276. https://doi.org/10.1039/c8ra09814j

Cao, D., Wang, Q., Zhu, S., Zhang, X., Li, Y., Cui, Y., Xue, Z., & Gao, S. (2021). Hydrothermal construction of flower-like MoS_2 on TiO_2 NTs for highly efficient environmental remediation and photocatalytic hydrogen evolution. *Separation and Purification Technology*, *265*, 118463. https://doi.org/10.1016/j.seppur.2021.118463

Cao, J., Zhou, J., Zhang, Y., & Liu, X. (2017). A clean and facile synthesis strategy of MoS 2 nanosheets grown on multi-wall CNTs for enhanced hydrogen evolution reaction performance. *Scientific Reports*, 1–8. https://doi.org/10.1038/s41598-017-09047-x

Chakrabarty, S., Mukherjee, A., & Basu, S. (2018). RGO-MoS_2 supported NiCo2O4 catalyst towards solar water splitting and dye degradation. *ACS Sustainable Chemistry & Engineering*, *6*(4), 5238–5247. https://doi.org/10.1021/acssuschemeng.7b04757

Chandrabose, G., Dey, A., Gaur, S. S., Pitchaimuthu, S., Jagadeesan, H., Braithwaite, N. S. J., Selvaraj, V., Kumar, V., & Krishnamurthy, S. (2021). Removal and degradation of mixed dye pollutants by integrated adsorption-photocatalysis technique using 2-D MoS_2/TiO_2 nanocomposite. *Chemosphere*, *279*, 130467. https://doi.org/10.1016/j.chemosphere.2021.130467

Chaudhary, N., Khanuja, M., & Islam, S. S. (2018). Highlights of research work SC. *Sensors and Actuators A: Physical*. https://doi.org/10.1016/j.sna.2018.05.008

Chen, H. J., Huang, J., Lei, X. L., Wu, M. S., Liu, G., Ouyang, C. Y., & Xu, B. (2013). Adsorption and diffusion of lithium on MoS_2 monolayer: The role of strain and concentration. *International Journal of Electrochemical Science*, *8*, 2196–2203.

Chen, Q., Zhao, C., Wang, Y., Chen, Y., Ma, Y., Chen, Z., Yu, J., Wu, Y., & He, Y. (2018). Synthesis of MoS_2/YVO_4 composite and its high photocatalytic performance in methyl orange degradation and H_2 evolution. *Solar Energy*, *171*, 426–434. https://doi.org/10.1016/j.solener.2018.06.112

Chen, S., Di, Y., Li, H., Wang, M., Jia, B., Xu, R., & Liu, X. (2021). Efficient photocatalytic dye degradation by flowerlike $MoS_2/SrFe_{12}O_{19}$ heterojunction under visible light. *Applied Surface Science*, *559*, 149855. https://doi.org/10.1016/j.apsusc.2021.149855

Chen, T., Yin, D., Zhao, F., Kyu, K. K., Liu, B., Chen, D., Huang, K., Deng, L. L., & Li, L. (2019). Fabrication of 2D heterojunction photocatalyst Co-g-C_3N_4/MoS_2 with enhanced solar-light-driven photocatalytic activity. *New Journal of Chemistry*, *43*, 463–473. https://doi.org/10.1039/c8nj04849e

Cravanzola, S., Cesano, F., Magnacca, G., Zecchina, A., & Scarano, D. (2016). Designing rGO/MoS_2 hybrid nanostructures for photocatalytic applications. *RSC Advances*, *6*, 59001–59008. https://doi.org/10.1039/c6ra08633k

Di, J., Xia, J., Ge, Y., Xu, L., Xu, H., Chen, J., He, M., & Li, H. (2014). Facile fabrication and enhanced visible light photocatalytic activity of few-layer MoS_2 coupled BiOBr microspheres. *Dalton Transactions*, *43*, 15429–15438. https://doi.org/10.1039/c4dt01652a

Drmosh, Q. A., Hezam, A., Hendi, A. H. Y., Qamar, M., Yamani, Z. H., & Byrappa, K. (2020). Ternary Bi_2S_3/MoS_2/TiO_2 with double Z-scheme configuration as high performance photocatalyst. *Applied Surface Science*, *499*. https://doi.org/10.1016/j.apsusc.2019.143938

Duphil, D., & Le, C. (2002). Chemical synthesis of molybdenum disulfide nanoparticles in an organic solution. *Journal of Materials Chemistry*, *12*, 2430–2432. https://doi.org/10.1039/b202162e

Fu, Y., Li, Z., Liu, Q., Yang, X., & Tang, H. (2017). Construction of carbon nitride and MoS $_2$ quantum dot 2D/0D hybrid photocatalyst: Direct Z – scheme mechanism for improved photocatalytic activity. *Chinese Journal of Catalysis*, *38*, 2160–2170. https://doi.org/10.1016/S1872-2067(17)62911-5

Gopika, M. S., & Bindhu, B. (2019). Preparation and characterization of few layered MoS_2 nano flakes. *International Journal of Recent Technology and Engineering*, *8*, 146–148. https://doi.org/10.35940/ijrte.B1027.0782S319

Goud, B. S., Koyyada, G., Jung, J. H., Reddy, G. R., Shim, J., Nam, N. D., & Vattikuti, S. V. P. (2020). Surface oxygen vacancy facilitated Z-scheme MoS_2/Bi_2O_3 heterojunction for enhanced visible-light driven photocatalysis-pollutant degradation and hydrogen production. *International Journal of Hydrogen Energy*, *45*, 18961–18975. https://doi.org/10.1016/j.ijhydene.2020.05.073

Guo, N., Li, H., Xu, X., & Yu, H. (2016). Hierarchical $Fe_{3\,4}$ @MoS_2/Ag_3 PO_4 magnetic nanocomposites: Enhanced and stable photocatalytic performance for water purification under visible light irradiation. *Applied Surface Science*, *389*, 227–239. https://doi.org/10.1016/j.apsusc.2016.07.099

Gupta, D., Chauhan, V., & Kumar, R. (2020). A comprehensive review on synthesis and applications of molybdenum disulfide (MoS) Material: Past and recent developments a comprehensive review on synthesis and applications of molybdenum disulfide (MoS_2) material: Past and recent developments. *Inorganic Chemistry Communications*, *121*, 108200. https://doi.org/10.1016/j.inoche.2020.108200

Han, W., Xia, Y., Yang, D., & Dong, A. (2021). Exfoliation of large-flake, few-layer MoS_2 nanosheets mediated by carbon nanotubes. *Chemical Communications*, *57*, 4400–4403. https://doi.org/10.1039/d1cc00673h

Harish, S., Bharathi, P., Prasad, P., Ramesh, R., Ponnusamy, S., Shimomura, M., Archana, J., & Navaneethan, M. (2021). Interface enriched highly interlaced layered MoS_2/NiS_2 nanocomposites for the photocatalytic degradation of rhodamine B dye. *RSC Advances*, *11*, 19283–19293. https://doi.org/10.1039/d1ra01941d

Hasija, V., Raizada, P., Sudhaik, A., Sharma, K., Kumar, A., Singh, P., Jonnalagadda, S. B., & Thakur, V. K. (2019). Recent advances in noble metal free doped graphitic carbon nitride based nanohybrids for photocatalysis of organic contaminants in water: A review. *Applied Materials Today*, *15*, 494–524. https://doi.org/10.1016/j.apmt.2019.04.003

He, Y., Ma, Z., & Junior, L. B. (2020). Distinctive binary g-C_3N_4/MoS_2 heterojunctions with highly efficient ultrasonic catalytic degradation for levofloxacin and methylene blue. *Ceramics International*, *46*, 12364–12372. https://doi.org/10.1016/j.ceramint.2020.01.287

He, Z., & Que, W. (2016). Molybdenum disulfide nanomaterials: Structures, properties, synthesis and recent progress on hydrogen evolution reaction. *Applied Materials Today*, *3*, 23–56. https://doi.org/10.1016/j.apmt.2016.02.001

Huang, H., Liu, C., Ou, H., Ma, T., & Zhang, Y. (2019). Self-sacrifice transformation for fabrication of type-I and type-II heterojunctions in hierarchical $Bi_xO_yI_z$/g-C_3N_4 for efficient visible-light photocatalysis. *Applied Surface Science*, *470*, 1101–1110. https://doi.org/10.1016/j.apsusc.2018.11.193

Ikram, M., Khan, M. I., Raza, A., Imran, M., Ul-Hamid, A., & Ali, S. (2020). Outstanding performance of silver-decorated MoS_2 nanopetals used as nanocatalyst for synthetic dye degradation. *Physica E: Low-Dimensional Systems Nanostructures*, *124*, 114246. https://doi.org/10.1016/j.physe.2020.114246

Jaleel, U. C. J. R., & Devi, K. R. S. (2020). Materials Statistical and experimental studies of MoS $_2$/g-C_3N_4/TiO_2: A ternary Z-scheme hybrid composite. *Journal of Materials Science*, *56*, 6922–6944. https://doi.org/10.1007/s10853-020-05695-z

Jaleel, U. C. J. R., Devi, K. R. S., Madhushree, R., & Pinheiro, D. (2021). Statistical and experimental studies of MoS_2/g-C_3N_4/TiO_2: A ternary Z-scheme hybrid composite. *Journal of Materials Science*, *56*, 6922–6944. https://doi.org/10.1007/s10853-020-05695-z

Jo, W. K., Lee, J. Y., & Selvam, N. C. S. (2016). Synthesis of MoS_2 nanosheets loaded ZnO-g-C_3N_4 nanocomposites for enhanced photocatalytic applications. *Chemical Engineering Journal*, *289*, 306–318. https://doi.org/10.1016/j.cej.2015.12.080

Khan, M. I., Hasan, M. S., Bhatti, K. A., Rizvi, H., Wahab, A., Rehman, S. U., Afzal, M. J., Nazneen, A., Fiaz Khan, M., Nazir, A., & Iqbal, M. (2020). Effect of Ni doping on the structural, optical and photocatalytic activity of MoS_2, prepared by Hydrothermal method. *Materials Research Express*, *7*. https://doi.org/10.1088/2053-1591/ab66f7

Kumar, S., Sharma, V., Bhattacharyya, K., & Krishnan, V. (2016). Synergetic effect of MoS_2-RGO doping to enhance the photocatalytic performance of ZnO nanoparticles. *New Journal of Chemistry*, *40*, 5185–5197. https://doi.org/10.1039/c5nj03595c

Lai, H., Ma, G., Shang, W., Chen, D., Yun, Y., Peng, X., & Xu, F. (2019). Multifunctional magnetic sphere-MoS_2@Au hybrid for surface-enhanced Raman scattering detection and visible light photo-Fenton degradation of aromatic dyes. *Chemosphere*, *223*, 465–473. https://doi.org/10.1016/j.chemosphere.2019.02.073

Li, M., Wang, D., Li, J., Pan, Z., Ma, H., Jiang, Y., & Tian, Z. (2016). Facile hydrothermal synthesis of MoS_2 nanosheets with controllable structures and enhanced catalytic performance for anthracene hydrogenation. *RSC Advances*, *6*, 71534–71542. https://doi.org/10.1039/c6ra16084k

Li, X. L., Ge, J. P., & Li, Y. D. (2004). Atmospheric pressure chemical vapor deposition: An alternative route to large-scale MoS_2 and WS2 inorganic fullerene-like nanostructures and nanoflowers. *Chemistry: A European Journal*, *10*, 6163–6171. https://doi.org/10.1002/chem.200400451

Li, X. L., & Zhu, H. (2015). Two-dimensional MoS_2: Properties, preparation, and applications. *Journal of Materiomics*, *1*, 33–44. https://doi.org/10.1016/j.jmat.2015.03.003

Li, Z., Meng, X., & Zhang, Z. (2018). Recent development on MoS_2-based photocatalysis: A review. *Journal of Photochemistry and Photobiology C: Photochemistry Reviews*, *35*, 39–55. https://doi.org/10.1016/j.jphotochemrev.2017.12.002

Liang, H., Yu, M., Guo, J., Zhan, R., Chen, J., Li, D., Zhang, L., & Niu, J. (2021). A novel vacancy-strengthened Z-scheme g-C_3N_4/Bp/MoS_2 composite for super-efficient visible-light photocatalytic degradation of ciprofloxacin. *Separation and Purification Technology*, *272*, 118891. https://doi.org/10.1016/j.seppur.2021.118891

Lin, Y. C., Zhang, W., Huang, J. K., Liu, K. K., Lee, Y. H., Liang, C. Te, Chu, C. W., & Li, L. J. (2012). Wafer-scale MoS_2 thin layers prepared by MoO_3 sulfurization. *Nanoscale*, *4*, 6637–6641. https://doi.org/10.1039/c2nr31833d

Liu, J., Zeng, Z., Cao, X., Lu, G., Wang, L., & Fan, Q. (2012). Preparation of MoS_2-polyvinylpyrrolidone nanocomposites for flexible nonvolatile rewritable memory devices with reduced graphene oxide electrodes, 1–6. https://doi.org/10.1002/smll.201200999

Liu, K. K., Zhang, W., Lee, Y. H., Lin, Y. C., Chang, M. T., Su, C. Y., Chang, C. S., Li, H., Shi, Y., Zhang, H., Lai, C. S., & Li, L. J. (2012). Growth of large-area and highly crystalline MoS_2 thin layers on insulating substrates. *Nano Letters*, *12*, 1538–1544. https://doi.org/10.1021/nl2043612

Liu, Y., Ren, L., Qi, X., Yang, L., Li, J., Wang, Y., & Zhong, J. (2014). Hydrothermal exfoliated molybdenum disulfide nanosheets as anode material for lithium ion batteries. *Journal of Energy Chemistry*, *23*, 207–212. https://doi.org/10.1016/S2095-4956(14)60137-6

Liu, Y., Yu, Y. X., & Zhang, W. De. (2013). MoS_2/CdS heterojunction with high photoelectrochemical activity for H2 evolution under visible light: The role of MoS_2. *The Journal of Physical Chemistry C*, *117*, 12949–12957. https://doi.org/10.1021/jp4009652

Liu, Y. D., Ren, L., Qi, X., Yang, L. W., Hao, G. L., Li, J., Wei, X. L., & Zhong, J. X. (2013). Preparation, characterization and photoelectrochemical property of ultrathin MoS_2 nanosheets via hydrothermal intercalation and exfoliation route. *Journal of Alloys and Compounds*, *571*, 37–42. https://doi.org/10.1016/j.jallcom.2013.03.031

Low, J., Yu, J., Jaroniec, M., Wageh, S., & Al-Ghamdi, A. A. (2017). Heterojunction Photocatalysts. *Advanced Materials*, *29*. https://doi.org/10.1002/adma.201601694

Lu, X., Jin, Y., Zhang, X., Xu, G., Wang, D., Lv, J., Zheng, Z., & Wu, Y. (2016). Controllable synthesis of graphitic C_3N_4/ultrathin MoS_2 nanosheet hybrid nanostructures with enhanced photocatalytic performance. *Dalton Transactions*, *45*, 15406–15414. https://doi.org/10.1039/c6dt02247b

Lukowski, M. A., Daniel, A. S., Meng, F., Forticaux, A., Li, L., & Jin, S. (2013). Enhanced hydrogen evolution catalysis from chemically exfoliated metallic MoS_2 nanosheets. *Journal of the American Chemical Society*, *135*, 10274–10277. https://doi.org/10.1021/ja404523s

McDaniel, H., Heil, P. E., Tsai, C. L., Kim, K., & Shim, M. (2011). Integration of type II nanorod heterostructures into photovoltaics. *ACS Nano*, *5*, 7677–7683. https://doi.org/10.1021/nn2029988

Mouloua, D., Kotbi, A., Deokar, G., Kaja, K., Marssi, M. El, Ali, M., Khakani, E. L., & Jouiad, M. (2021). Recent progress in the synthesis of MoS_2 thin films for sensing, photovoltaic and plasmonic applications: A review. *Materials (Basel)*, *14*(12), 3283.

Muralikrishna, S., Manjunath, K., Samrat, D., Reddy, V., Ramakrishnappa, T., & Nagaraju, D. H. (2015). RSC Advances electrocatalytic hydrogen evolution reaction. *RSC Advances*, *5*, 89389–89396. https://doi.org/10.1039/C5RA18855E

Nagaraju, G., Tharamani, C. N., Chandrappa, G. T., & Livage, J. (2007). Hydrothermal synthesis of amorphous MoS_2 nanofiber bundles via acidification of ammonium heptamolybdate tetrahydrate. *Nanoscale Research Letters*, *2*, 461–468. https://doi.org/10.1007/s11671-007-9087-z

Nayak, S., Swain, G., & Parida, K. (2019). Enhanced photocatalytic activities of RhB degradation and H2 evolution from in situ formation of the electrostatic heterostructure MoS_2/NiFe LDH nanocomposite through the Z-scheme mechanism via p–n heterojunctions. *ACS Applied Materials & Interfaces*, *11*, 20923–20942. https://doi.org/10.1021/acsami.9b06511

Panigrahi, P. K., & Pathak, A. (2011). A novel route for the synthesis of nanotubes and fullerene-like nanostructures of molybdenum disulfide. *Materials Research Bulletin*, *46*, 2240–2246. https://doi.org/10.1016/j.materresbull.2011.09.003

Paul, K. K., Sreekanth, N., Biroju, R. K., Narayanan, T. N., & Giri, P. K. (2018). Solar light driven photoelectrocatalytic hydrogen evolution and dye degradation by metal-free few-layer MoS_2 nanoflower/TiO2(B) nanobelts heterostructure. *Solar Energy Materials and Solar Cells*, *185*, 364–374. https://doi.org/10.1016/j.solmat.2018.05.056

Peng, K., Wang, H., Li, X., Wang, J., Xu, L., Gao, H., & Niu, M. (2019). Applied clay science one-step hydrothermal growth of MoS_2 nanosheets/CdS nanoparticles heterostructures on montmorillonite for enhanced visible light photocatalytic activity. *Applied Clay Science*, *175*, 86–93. https://doi.org/10.1016/j.clay.2019.04.007

Peng, W. C., & Li, X. Y. (2014). Synthesis of MoS_2/g-C_3N_4 as a solar light-responsive photocatalyst for organic degradation. *Catalysis Communications*, *49*, 63–67. https://doi.org/10.1016/j.catcom.2014.02.008

Prabhakar Vattikuti, S. V., Byon, C., Venkata Reddy, C., Venkatesh, B., & Shim, J. (2015). Synthesis and structural characterization of MoS_2 nanospheres and nanosheets using solvothermal method. *Journal of Materials Science*, *50*, 5024–5038. https://doi.org/10.1007/s10853-015-9051-8

Qin, N., Xiong, J., Liang, R., Liu, Y., Zhang, S., Li, Y., Li, Z., & Wu, L. (2016). Highly efficient photocatalytic H_2 evolution over MoS_2/CdS-TiO2 nanofibers prepared by an electrospinning mediated photodeposition method. *Applied Catalysis B: Environmental*. https://doi.org/10.1016/j.apcatb.2016.09.040

Radisavljevic, B., Radenovic, A., Brivio, J., Giacometti, V., & Kis, A. (2011). Single-layer MoS_2 transistors. *Nature Nanotechnology*, *6*, 147–150. https://doi.org/10.1038/nnano.2010.279

Rani, A., Singh, K., Patel, A. S., Chakraborti, A., Kumar, S., Ghosh, K., & Sharma, P. (2019). Visible light driven photocatalysis of organic dyes using SnO_2 decorated MoS_2 nanocomposites. *Chemical Physics Letters*, 136874. https://doi.org/10.1016/j.cplett.2019.136874

Rao Akshatha, S., Sreenivasa, S., Parashuram, L., Raghu, M. S., Yogesh Kumar, K., & Madhu Chakrapani Rao, T. (2020). Visible-light-induced photochemical hydrogen evolution and degradation of crystal violet dye by interwoven layered MoS_2/Wurtzite ZnS heterostructure photocatalyst. *ChemistrySelect*, *5*, 6918–6926. https://doi.org/10.1002/slct.202001914

Raza, A., Ikram, M., Aqeel, M., Imran, M., Ul, A., Nadeem, K., & Salamat, R. (2020). Enhanced industrial dye degradation using Co doped in chemically exfoliated MoS_2 nanosheets. *Applied Nanoscience*, *10*, 1535–1544. https://doi.org/10.1007/s13204-019-01239-3

Sadhanala, H. K., Senapati, S., Harika, K. V., Nanda, K. K., & Gedanken, A. (2018). Green synthesis of MoS_2 nanoflowers for efficient degradation of methylene blue and crystal violet dyes under natural sun light conditions. *New Journal of Chemistry*, *42*, 14318–14324. https://doi.org/10.1039/c8nj01731j

Sharma, P., Singh, M. K., & Mehata, M. S. (2021). Sunlight-driven MoS_2 nanosheets mediated degradation of dye (crystal violet) for wastewater treatment. *Journal of Molecular Structure*, *1249*, 131651. https://doi.org/10.1016/j.molstruc.2021.131651

Taiwo, I., Odunayo, A., Adedokun, O., & Mokhotjwa, S. (2020). Recent advances on the preparation and electrochemical analysis of MoS_2-based materials for supercapacitor applications: A mini-review. *Materials Today Communications*, *25*, 101664. https://doi.org/10.1016/j.mtcomm.2020.101664

Tama, A. M., Das, S., Dutta, S., Bhuyan, M. D. I., Islam, M. N., & Basith, M. A. (2019). MoS_2 nanosheet incorporated α-Fe_2O_3/ZnO nanocomposite with enhanced photocatalytic dye degradation and hydrogen production ability. *RSC Advances*, *9*, 40357–40367. https://doi.org/10.1039/c9ra07526g

Tang, G., Chen, Y., Yin, J., & Cai, K. (2017). Preparation, characterization and properties of MoS_2 nanosheets via a microwave-assisted wet-chemical route. *Ceramics International*, *44*(5), 5336–5340. https://doi.org/10.1016/j.ceramint.2017.12.152

Tang, Q., An, X., Zhou, J., Lan, H., Liu, H., & Qu, J. (2020). One-step exfoliation of polymeric g-C_3N_4 by atmospheric oxygen doping for photocatalytic persulfate activation. *Journal of Colloid and Interface Science*, *579*, 455–462. https://doi.org/10.1016/j.jcis.2020.06.064

Tao, L., Long, H., Zhou, B., Yu, S. F., Lau, S. P., Chai, Y., Fung, K. H., Tsang, Y. H., Yao, J., & Xu, D. (2014). Preparation and characterization of few-layer MoS_2 nanosheets and their good nonlinear optical responses in the PMMA matrix. *Nanoscale*, *6*, 9713–9719. https://doi.org/10.1039/c4nr02664k

Theerthagiri, J., Senthil, R. A., Senthilkumar, B., Reddy, A., & Madhavan, J. (2017). Recent advances in MoS 2 nanostructured materials for energy and environmental applications—A review. *Journal of Solid State Chemistry*, *252*, 43–71. https://doi.org/10.1016/j.jssc.2017.04.041

Tian, S., Zhang, X., & Zhang, Z. (2020). Capacitive deionization with MoS_2/g-C_3N_4 electrodes. *Desalination*, *479*. https://doi.org/10.1016/j.desal.2020.114348

Ullah, H., Khan, Z., Nasir, J. A., Balkan, T., Butler, I. S., Kaya, S., & Rehman, Z. ur. (2021). Green synthesis of mesoporous MoS_2 nanoflowers for efficient photocatalytic degradation of Congo red dye. *Journal of Coordination Chemistry*, *74*, 2302–2314. https://doi.org/10.1080/00958972.2021.1962523

Vattikuti, A. S. V. P., & Byon, C. (2016). Bi2S3 nanorods embedded with MoS_2 nanosheets composite for photodegradation of phenol red under visible light irradiation. *Superlattices and Microstructures*, *100*, 514–525. https://doi.org/10.1016/j.spmi.2016.10.012

Vattikuti, A. S. V. P., & Byon, C. (2017). Hydrothermally synthesized ternary heterostructured $MoS_2/Al_2O_3/g\text{-}C_3N_4$ photocatalyst. *Materials Research Bulletin*. https://doi.org/10.1016/j.materresbull.2017.03.008

Vattikuti, A. S. V. P., Byon, C., & Venkata, C. (2015). Synthesis and structural characterization of MoS_2 nanospheres and nanosheets using solvothermal method. *Journal of Materials Science*. https://doi.org/10.1007/s10853-015-9051-8

Voiry, D., Mohite, A., & Chhowalla, M. (2015). Phase engineering of transition metal dichalcogenides. *Chemical Society Reviews*, *44*, 2702–2712. https://doi.org/10.1039/c5cs00151j

Wang, J., Wei, B., Xu, L., Gao, H., Sun, W., & Che, J. (2016). Multilayered MoS_2 coated TiO_2 hollow spheres for efficient photodegradation of phenol under visible light irradiation. *Materials Letters*, *179*, 42–46. https://doi.org/10.1016/j.matlet.2016.05.032

Wang, S., Li, D., Sun, C., Yang, S., Guan, Y., & He, H. (2014). Synthesis and characterization of $g\text{-}C_3N_4/Ag_3VO_4$ composites with significantly enhanced visible-light photocatalytic activity for triphenylmethane dye degradation. *Applied Catalysis B: Environmental*, *144*, 885–892. https://doi.org/10.1016/j.apcatb.2013.08.008

Wang, T., Chen, S., Pang, H., Xue, H., & Yu, Y. (2017). MoS_2-based nanocomposites for electrochemical energy storage. *Advanced Science*, *4*. https://doi.org/10.1002/advs.201600289

Wang, W., Zhang, K., Qiao, Z., Li, L., Liu, P., & Yang, Y. (2014). Influence of surfactants on the synthesis of MoS_2 catalysts and their activities in the hydrodeoxygenation of 4-methylphenol. *Industrial & Engineering Chemistry Research*, *53*(25), 10301–10309.

Wang, X., Feng, H., Wu, Y., Jiao, L., Wang, X., Feng, H., Wu, Y., & Jiao, L. (2013). Controlled synthesis of highly crystalline MoS_2 flakes by chemical vapor deposition. *Journal of the American Chemical Society*, *135*(14), 5304–5307. https://doi.org/10.1021/ja4013485

Wang, Y., Shang, X., Shen, J., Zhang, Z., Wang, D., Lin, J., Wu, J. C. S., Fu, X., Wang, X., & Li, C. (2020). Direct and indirect Z-scheme heterostructure-coupled photosystem enabling cooperation of CO_2 reduction and H2O oxidation. *Nature Communications*, *11*, 1–11. https://doi.org/10.1038/s41467-020-16742-3

Wang, Z., & Mi, B. (2017). Environmental applications of 2D molybdenum disulfide (MoS_2) nanosheets. *Environmental Science & Technology*, *51*, 8229–8244. https://doi.org/10.1021/acs.est.7b01466

Xu, J., Tang, H., Zhang, K., Zhang, H., Li, C., & Province, J. (2014). Synthesis and tribological properties of flower-like MoS_2 microspheres. *Ceramics International*, *201440*(8), 11575–11580.

Xu, Q., Zhang, L., Cheng, B., Fan, J., & Yu, J. (2020). S-scheme heterojunction photocatalyst. *Chem*, *6*, 1543–1559. https://doi.org/10.1016/j.chempr.2020.06.010

Xu, Q., Zhang, L., Yu, J., Wageh, S., Al-Ghamdi, A. A., & Jaroniec, M. (2018). Direct Z-scheme photocatalysts: Principles, synthesis, and applications. *Materials Today*, *21*, 1042–1063. https://doi.org/10.1016/j.mattod.2018.04.008

Xue, B., Jiang, H., Sun, T., Mao, F., & Wu, J. (2018). One-step synthesis of MoS $_2$/g-C_3N_4 nanocomposites with highly enhanced photocatalytic activity. *Materials Letters*, *228*, 475–478. https://doi.org/10.1016/j.matlet.2018.06.094

Yang, F., Zhang, Z., Wang, Y., Xu, M., Zhao, W., Yan, J., & Chen, C. (2017). Facile synthesis of nano-MoS_2 and its visible light photocatalytic property. *Materials Research Bulletin*, *87*, 119–122. https://doi.org/10.1016/j.materresbull.2016.11.029

Ye, L., Xu, H., Zhang, D., & Chen, S. (2014). Synthesis of bilayer MoS_2 nanosheets by a facile hydrothermal method and their methyl orange adsorption capacity. *Materials Research Bulletin*, *55*, 221–228. https://doi.org/10.1016/j.materresbull.2014.04.025

Yuan, Y., Shen, P., Li, Q., Chen, G., Zhang, H., Zhu, L., & Zou, B. (2017). Excellent photocatalytic performance of few-layer MoS_2/graphene hybrids. *Journal of Alloys and Compounds*, *700*, 12–17. https://doi.org/10.1016/j.jallcom.2017.01.027

Zeng, Y., Guo, N., Li, H., Wang, Q., Xu, X., Yu, Y., Han, X., & Yu, H. (2019). Construction of flower-like MoS_2/Ag_2S/Ag Z-scheme photocatalysts with enhanced visible-light photocatalytic activity for water purification. *Science of the Total Environment*, *659*, 20–32. https://doi.org/10.1016/j.scitotenv.2018.12.333

Zhang, B., Shi, H., Hu, X., Wang, Y., Liu, E., & Fan, J. (2020). A novel S-scheme MoS_2/$CdIn_2S_4$ flower-like heterojunctions with enhanced photocatalytic degradation and H_2 evolution activity. *Journal of Physics D: Applied Physics*, *53*. https://doi.org/10.1088/1361-6463/ab7563

Zhang, R. Z., Chen, Q. W., Lei, Y. X., & Zhou, J. P. (2019). Growth of MoS_2 nanosheets on TiO2/g-C3N4 nanocomposites to enhance the visible-light photocatalytic ability. *Journal of Materials Science: Materials in Electronics*, *30*, 5393–5403. https://doi.org/10.1007/s10854-019-00832-0

Zhang, W., Xiao, X., Li, Y., Zeng, X., Zheng, L., & Wan, C. (2016). Liquid-exfoliation of layered Mo $_2$ for enhancing photocatalytic activity of TiO_2/g-C_3N_4 photocatalyst and DFT study. *Applied Surface Science*, *389*, 496–506. https://doi.org/10.1016/j.apsusc.2016.07.154

Zhang, W., Zhang, P., & Wei, G. (2015). Synthesis and sensor applications of MoS_2-based nanocomposites. *Nanoscale*, 18364–18378. https://doi.org/10.1039/c5nr06121k

Zhang, X., Wu, J., Williams, G. R., Yang, Y., Niu, S., Qian, Q., & Zhu, L. M. (2019). Dual-responsive molybdenum disulfide/copper sulfide-based delivery systems for enhanced chemo-photothermal therapy. *Journal of Colloid and Interface Science*, *539*, 433–441. https://doi.org/10.1016/j.jcis.2018.12.072

Zhang, X. H., Wang, C., Xue, M. Q., Lin, B. C., Ye, X., Lei, W. N., Province, J., & Province, J. (2016). Hydrothermal synthesis and characterization of ultrathin MoS_2 nanosheets. *Chalcogenide Letters*, *13*, 27–34.

Zhang, Y., Ju, P., Hao, L., Zhai, X., Jiang, F., & Sun, C. (2021). Novel Z-scheme MoS_2/Bi_2WO_6 heterojunction with highly enhanced photocatalytic activity under visible light irradiation. *Journal of Alloys and Compounds*, *854*, 157224. https://doi.org/10.1016/j.jallcom.2020.157224

Zhao, G., Hou, J., Wu, Y., He, J., & Hao, X. (2015a). Preparation of 2D MoS_2/graphene heterostructure through a monolayer intercalation method and its application as an optical modulator in pulsed laser generation, 1–6. https://doi.org/10.1002/adom.201500012

Zhao, Z., Sun, Y., Dong, F., Zhang, Y., & Zhao, H. (2015b). Template synthesis of carbon self-doped g-C_3N_4 with enhanced visible to near-infrared absorption and photocatalytic performance. *RSC Advances*. https://doi.org/10.1039/c5ra03433g

Zhou, J., Lan, X., Ren, P., Zhang, Q., Song, Y., & Chen, X. (2011). Synthesis and characterization of flower-sphere MoS_2. *Materials Science Forum*, *695*, 429–432. https://doi.org/10.4028/www.scientific.net/MSF.695.429

Zhou, Y., Fan, X., Zhang, G., & Dong, W. (2019). Fabricating MoS_2 nanoflakes photoanode with unprecedented high photoelectrochemical performance and multi-pollutants degradation test for water treatment. *Chemical Engineering Journal*, *356*, 1003–1013. https://doi.org/10.1016/j.cej.2018.09.097

Zhu, C., Zhang, L., Jiang, B., Zheng, J., Hu, P., Li, S., Wu, M., & Wu, W. (2016). Fabrication of Z-scheme Ag_3PO_4/MoS_2 composites with enhanced photocatalytic activity and stability for organic pollutant degradation. *Applied Surface Science*, *377*, 99–108. https://doi.org/10.1016/j.apsusc.2016.03.143

6 Integrated Biomedical Waste Management

Critical Analysis on Sustainable Circular Economy

Sudipti Arora, Saurabh Dhakad, Devanshi Sutaria, and Sonika Saxena

6.1 INTRODUCTION

The global waste generation dynamics have been altered due to the COVID-19 pandemic, necessitating specific attention to make a solid waste management plan. Policymakers must also respond dynamically to unforeseen changes in waste composition and amounts. Further, the COVID-19 pandemic has demonstrated the importance of waste management services. Safely disposing of and

DOI: 10.1201/9781003499695-6

treating COVID-19–related biological waste and managing waste treatment plants is becoming increasingly difficult. Due to COVID-19, the demand for medical equipment has dramatically increased, especially during diagnosis and treatment, resulting in a considerable amount of solid and medical waste generated worldwide (Choudhury et al., 2022). Alongside this is a vital issue of municipal solid waste along with the handling of infectious medical waste (IMW). Considering that inappropriate IMW management can result in a high disease burden, it is an important aspect of controlling contagious disease (Madsen et al., 2020). During an outbreak, many types of medical and hazardous waste are generated, including infected masks, gloves, other protective equipment, and non-infected goods (UNEP, 2020). Most waste-handling personnel must be adequately trained, putting them at significant risk of complications. People in home quarantines frequently discard their household waste in the same bin as their contaminated face masks, tissue paper, and other contaminated waste, posing a risk of disease transmission to municipal personnel and rag pickers who collect garbage. As a result, any delay or inability to handle biohazardous waste can result in significant and irreversible illness and mortality. The current chapter interprets existing worldwide biomedical waste management procedures and provides unique insights into the pandemic's impact on biomedical, plastic, and food waste generation. The chapter also presents the Biomedical Waste (BMW) management scenario in India, Lebanon, Bangladesh, and China. The chapter emphasizes the issues faced by the waste management sector during the pandemic crisis and points out the existing system gaps, thus laying the foundation for Chapters 7 to 10.

6.2 COVID-19 AND SOLID WASTE MANAGEMENT

6.2.1 Waste Management Challenges

The government has encountered a massive problem in dealing with the pandemic (COVID-19) crisis due to the present infrastructural facilities and insufficient safety equipment. Multiple testing facilities, rapid adjustments and improvisations in medical standards, and public policy changes have been formed to meet the present public health concerns (UNEP, 2020). To combat the spread of the SARS-CoV-2 virus, government agencies employed total lockdown, social distancing in public areas, self-quarantine for affected persons, and the use of personal protective equipment such as masks and gloves. As a result, garbage creation and management patterns have radically changed. Solid trash was handled by sanitary staff and sent to waste management centres before COVID-19. The waste emitted, however, is now classified as hazardous in nature and may include infectious organisms needing separate handling, treatment, and disposal facilities due to COVID-19 (Mallapur, 2020). COVID-19 waste (CW) can contaminate municipal garbage if it is not adequately disposed of, posing a risk of transmission to sanitary handlers as well as the public at large (UNEP, 2020). Due to the conditions that arose during the epidemic, governments have focused on and given special attention to waste management systems and treatment facilities for CW.

6.2.2 Waste Collection

To avoid contamination, waste bins should not be placed in public areas because more people will gather and use the same containers. Waste should be labelled as COVID-19 waste while it is delivered to common biomedical waste treatment facilities (CBWTFs) (CPCB guidelines, 2020). Waste collectors should receive proper PPE while collecting garbage from COVID-19 patients, hospitals, and laboratories. For detailed specifications regarding sources and categorization of biomedical wastes, colour coding, and type of container for BMW, refer to Chapters 7, 8, and 9 (BMW Rule, 2016).

6.2.3 Waste Sorting, Segregation, and Storage

Before the final disposal of solid waste, garbage must be separated and sorted. After collection, COVID-19 trash should be isolated from non-infectious medical waste such as paper, cardboard, and food scraps. The collected biomedical waste should be labelled with the waste type, generating site, and generation date before being transported from the generation site (BMW Rule, 2016). Following separation, each waste category should be placed in its own bag, with its top appropriately covered to prevent liquid waste from leaking out and contaminating the storage surface (BMW Rule, 2016) (refer to Chapters 7, 8, and 9).

6.2.4 Transportation

All COVID-19–contaminated waste products should be sealed before shipment with the proper barcode and record. For safe transportation, a proper transfer route; a dedicated, qualified driver; and a separate vehicle should be provided (BMW Rule, 2016) (refer to Chapters 7, 8 , and 9). It is not advisable to travel in busy regions or during rush hour. COVID-19 garbage should be collected by a waste collector with sufficient training.

6.2.5 Waste Processing, Treatment, and Final Disposal

The principal ways of dealing with COVID-19 waste are chemical treatment, autoclaving, and incineration. COVID-19 waste should be disposed of quickly after arriving at a disposal facility. If the trash load is large, the transported waste material can be temporarily held in a separate location designated for COVID-19 garbage for up to 12 hours (People's Republic of China Ministry of Ecology and Environment, 2020). For detailed specifications regarding waste processing, treatment, and final disposal of BMW, refer to Chapters 7, 8, and 9. Figure 6.1 describes the proper mechanism for integrated biomedical waste management.

6.3 PLASTIC WASTE MANAGEMENT AND THE ROLE OF THE CIRCULAR ECONOMY

Plastic demand for packaging is expected to rise by 40%, while demand for other applications, such as medical use, is expected to rise by 17% (Silva et al., 2021). Polyethylene terephthalate (PET) caps and polypropylene (PP) bottles should be prioritized for recycling. The recycling instructions should be clearly displayed on the packaging to make recycling easy. Many firms are experiencing a surge in business during COVID-19, but to maintain their environmentally friendly reputation, they must create packaging with sustainability as the primary priority, which necessitates paying attention to all components. Plastics cannot be completely eliminated from daily life. However, in some cases, it is possible to replace them. As an example, consider using reusable paper or cloth bags. Micro-algae–based bioplastics are made from biosynthesised materials and require 17% less energy to produce. Biopolymers include polyhydroxyalkanoates (PHAs), polyhydroxy butyrate (PHBs), and polylactic acids (PLAs), among others (Roy & Choudhury, 2022; Anjum et al., 2016).

6.4 CIRCULAR ECONOMY DURING COVID-19 AND BEYOND

The circular economy isn't just a theory; the concepts are still being used to assist us in dealing with the epidemic today. Manufacturing and

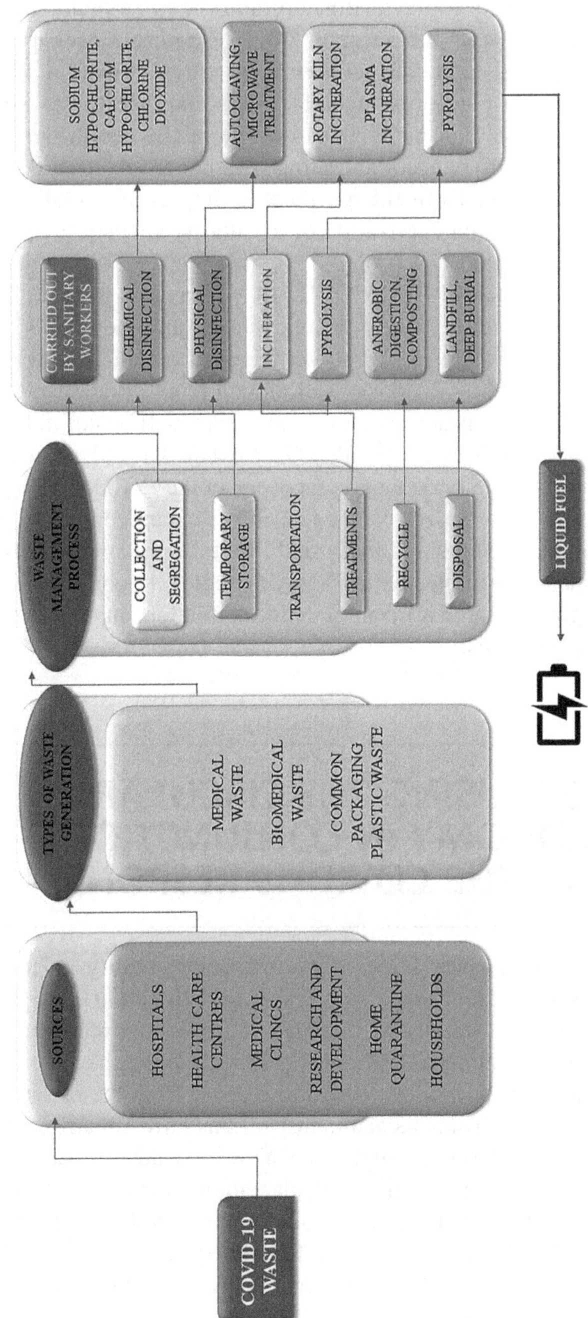

FIGURE 6.1 Mechanism of integrated medical waste management.

supply-chain bottlenecks in the healthcare industry in circular innovation have been pushed. Despite the surge in single-use plastic packaging as a result of quarantine-related home deliveries and worries linked with reused materials, responsible packaging manufacturers continue to develop sustainable and recyclable consumer items outside of the health sector. The food and beverage industry is collaborating with nonprofits to reroute extra food to people in need. Even though these examples are small and targeted, they show a greater realization of circularity's worth, both during and shortly after the crisis.

For example, to recover from COVID-19, Amsterdam became the first municipality to use the doughnut economics model and the circular 2020–2025 strategy. The new model and strategy have a specific goal of reducing food waste by half by 2030, as well as enforcing strict sustainability standards. By 2030, the usage of new raw materials will be cut in half, and construction tenders will be eliminated. Green deals have also been established as essential pillars of economic recovery in the European Union and South Korea, utilizing regenerative models and circular economy concepts. Circularity may be implemented today and in the future at all levels, from cleaning face masks to implementing SMART regional policies and strategies that maximize resource utilization, reduce pollution, and open up many commercial opportunities.

6.5 USING THE CIRCULAR ECONOMY IN CONJUNCTION WITH THE COVID-19 RESPONSE

In the long run, the answer is clear: post-pandemic reality must include resilience, decarbonization, and a sustainable growth path. Green stimulus packages outperformed traditional stimulus packages in a recent academic paper that examined numerous stimulus packages since the financial crisis. Given the amount of money needed to recover from the crisis and the growing number of governments and industries that have already committed to greening their industries through their nationally determined contributions and related climate mitigation and adaptation reforms, any COVID-19 stimulus should help countries achieve their medium- to long-term development goals. Many of the same ideas of a functional transition to the circular economy are required to build a system that survives unanticipated pressures rather than buckling under them.

6.6 WORLDWIDE SCENARIO OF MEDICAL WASTE MANAGEMENT DURING COVID-19: CASE STUDIES

6.6.1 India

COVID-19 impacts the most populous cities, such as Delhi, Mumbai, Bangalore, Chennai, and Hyderabad. According to data released by NDTV on September 18, 2020, the country produces a significant volume of COVID-19–related biological waste (over 100 tonnes per day). Maharashtra is responsible for roughly 17% of the total COVID-19–related BMW. The national daily garbage generation rate has risen to roughly 850 tonnes daily. The national daily garbage generation rate has risen to roughly 850 tonnes daily. The existence of 198 CBMWFs and 225 captive incinerators needed to be increased to dispose of 700 tonnes of garbage each day. However, the government has developed different standard operating procedures and revised existing rules and guidelines to combat this major problem in a timely manner (Goswami et al., 2021).

6.6.2 Lebanon

COVID-19 infections are on the rise in Lebanon, with over 252,000 cases and 1906 deaths documented as of January 17, 2021. In Lebanon, a comparable increase in the creation of medical waste is projected. The COVID-19 pandemic in Lebanon adds to the difficulty of managing trash created by households (MSW) and healthcare facilities. Due to technological, operational, economic, and/or financial constraints, Lebanon already needs more suitable healthcare and MSW management standards, and it is particularly vulnerable to the COVID-19 pandemic, which brings new risks and problems. COVID-19–related infectious healthcare waste accounted for 5 – 20% of overall infectious healthcare waste in Lebanon, with an estimated monthly average of 39,035 kg (1.3 tonnes) daily. According to the findings, the amount of isolated infectious medical waste has increased dramatically with the rising number of confirmed COVID-19 cases, which more than doubled after August 2020 and continues to rise. However, due to Lebanon's financial and economic crises, which also hampered the execution of a comprehensive healthcare waste management plan, total infectious medical waste in 2020 will be lower than in prior years (Maalouf & Maalouf, 2021).

6.6.3 Bangladesh

In Bangladesh, several national guidelines covering important issues related to the MWM system were formulated during the pandemic, which is commendable. During this pandemic, Bangladesh also published an impact assessment (IA) framework. However, no evidence of its implementation could be found. As a result, taking the initiative to implement this IA framework is required. Policymakers will be able to identify the gaps impeding the implementation of MWM policy tools and guidelines. This will allow them to take appropriate corrective actions to improve the MWM system by increasing preparedness and capacity for any potential future situations, such as a pandemic that overwhelms the MW situation in Bangladesh (Barua & Hossain, 2021).

6.6.4 China

The COVID-19 epidemic has considerably increased the daily output of medical waste in China, putting the country's medical waste disposal system to the test. Unlike conventional trash and garbage, medical waste that is left untreated or incompletely treated not only pollutes the environment but also causes illnesses and puts people's health at risk. Faced with challenges, the Chinese government developed a medical waste management policy and an epidemic response plan, which offers policy assurance for the standardized disposal of epidemic medical waste. By building new centralized disposal centres and adding mobile disposal facilities, China has improved the capacity of medical waste disposal in various locations. In the fight against COVID-19, China has made significant progress, and the strain on medical waste disposal has been lifted to some extent. The global epidemic situation, on the other hand, is dire. The prevention and control of epidemic situations are linked to the proper and safe disposal of medical waste. China's approach to medical waste disposal in the specific situation of COVID-19 can provide guidance for other countries dealing with medical waste disposal (Su et al., 2021).

6.7 CONCLUSIONS

The escalating impact of the COVID-19 pandemic underscores the critical need for effective global waste management, particularly regarding household and medical waste. Urgent action is required to inform the public about proper disposal methods for the surging volume of PPE, masks, and sanitizers. To address this, robust, long-term solid waste management plans are imperative, focusing on separating waste at its source. The incineration of residual waste at high temperatures aligns with the United Nations Environment Program's goal of sustainable waste management and preventing COVID-19 spread. Enforcing stringent laws is pivotal for successful waste management, averting disasters, and unlocking energy and financial resources. Future research should prioritize eco-friendly, biodegradable medical equipment to advance sustainability, reducing environmental costs in our pursuit of responsible production and consumption.

REFERENCES

Anjum, A., Zuber, M., Zia, K. M., Noreen, A., Anjum, M. N., & Tabasum, S. (2016). Microbial production of polyhydroxyalkanoates (PHAs) and its copolymers: A review of recent advancements. *International Journal of Biological Macromolecules*, *89*, 161–174.

Barua, U., & Hossain, D. (2021). A review of the medical waste management system at Covid-19 situation in Bangladesh. *Journal of Material Cycles and Waste Management*, *23*(6), 2087–2100.

Bio-Medical Waste Management (Principal) Rules. (2016). *Published in the Gazette of India, extraordinary, part II, section 3, sub-section (i)*. Government of India Ministry of Environment, Forest and Climate Change.

Choudhury, M., Sahoo, S., Samanta, P., Tiwari, A., Tiwari, A., Chadha, U., & Chakravorty, A. (2022). COVID-19: An accelerator for global plastic consumption and its implications. *Journal of Environmental and Public Health, 2022*. https://doi.org/10.1155/2022/1066350

Goswami, M., Goswami, P. J., Nautiyal, S., & Prakash, S. (2021). Challenges and actions to the environmental management of Bio-Medical Waste during COVID-19 pandemic in India.*Heliyon*, *7*(3), e06313.

Maalouf, A., & Maalouf, H. (2021). Impact of COVID-19 pandemic on medical waste management in Lebanon. *Waste Management & Research*, 0734242X211003970.

Madsen, A. M., Frederiksen, M. W., Bjerregaard, M., & Tendal, K. (2020). Measures to reduce the exposure of waste collection workers to handborne and airborne microorganisms and inflammogenic dust. *Waste Management*, *101*, 241–249.

Mallapur, C. (2020). Sanitation workers at risk from discarded medical waste related to COVID-19. *IndiaSpend*. Retrieved April 26, 2020, from https://www.indiaspend.com/sanitation-workers-at-risk-from-discarded-medical-waste-related-tocovid-19/

Revision, C. P. C. B. (2020). *Guidelines for handling, treatment and disposal of waste generated during treatment/diagnosis/quarantine of COVID-19 Patients*. Retrieved July 1. https://cpcb.nic.in/uploads/Projects/Bio-Medical-Waste/BMW-GUIDELINES-COVID_1.pdf

Roy, P., & Choudhury, M. (2022). Bioeconomy and green plastic production. In C. Baskar, S. Ramakrishna & A. Daniela La Rosa (Eds.), *Encyclopedia of green materials*. Springer. https://doi.org/10.1007/978-981-16-4921-9_189-1

Silva, A. L. P., Prata, J. C., Walker, T. R., Duarte, A. C., Ouyang, W., Barcelò, D., & Rocha-Santos, T. (2021). Increased plastic pollution due to COVID-19 pandemic: Challenges and recommendations. *Chemical Engineering Journal*, *405*, 126683.

Su, M., Wang, Q., & Li, R. (2021). How to dispose of medical waste caused by COVID-19? A case study of China. *International Journal of Environmental Research and Public Health*, *18*(22), 12127.

UNESCAP. (2018). *Closing the loop: Unlocking an inclusive circular economy approach*. Stakeholder Workshop in Pune, United Nations ESCAP, India. Retrieved July 5, 2020, from https://www.unescap.org/sites/default/files/Pune%20Workshop_Report_FINAL.pdf

UNESCAP. (2018). *Closing the loop: Unlocking an inclusive circular economy approach*. Stakeholder Workshop in Bangkok, United Nations ESCAP, Thailand. Retrieved July 5, 2020, from https://www.unescap.org/sites/default/files/Closing%20the%20Loop%20Bangkok%20Workshop_Final%20Report.pdf

Waste management an essential public service in the fight to beat COVID-19. https://www.unep.org/news-and-stories/press-release/waste-management-essential-public-service-fight-beat-covid-19

7 Biomedical Waste Management

Critical Analysis of Occupational Safety and Concerns

Nishu Mittal, Tsering Angmo, Shweta Rajpal, Kanwarpal S Dhugga, and Pallavi Gahlot

7.1 INTRODUCTION

Biomedical waste (BMW) refers to wastes generated from (Tenglikar et al., 2012) biological resources or laboratory waste where research, diagnosis, and prevention of human and animal diseases are carried out. Waste remains a complex problem for human societies due to its negative impact on the environment, socio-economic stability, and public health (Song et al., 2021). Unsafe medical waste disposal and inadequate management increase public health crises (Minoglou et al., 2017). Healthcare without Harm (HCWH) analysed

DOI: 10.1201/9781003499695-7

that the healthcare industry is the world's fifth-largest source of greenhouse gases (GHGs), accounting for approximately 4.4% of global net emissions (Karliner et al., 2019). In the COVID-19 scenario, some countries are expected to generate high volumes of medical waste (Choudhury et al., 2022). Improper management and increased unsafe handling of medical waste during the pandemic can pose an immediate danger to people and the environment (Peng et al., 2020). The data collected by the World Health Organization (WHO) show that new infectious diseases like HIV, hepatitis B, and hepatitis C are mainly transmitted through contaminated surgical objects, leading to approximately 32%, 40%, and 5% of total new infections, respectively. The sustainable and safe disposal of biomedical waste is a global concern due to its environmental and human health dangers. Primary biomedical waste sources include hospitals, nursing homes, medical clinics, testing laboratories, pharmaceuticals, and dispensaries.

Occupational safety and health is identified as the discipline dealing with the prevention of work-related injuries and diseases and the protection and promotion of workers' health. It aims to improve working conditions and the environment. The pandemic has made the global community realize the importance of considering occupational safety issues and implementing policies for safeguarding the environment and public health. The present chapter focuses on the directive policies, generation, segregation, and management of BMW's regulatory framework regarding safe handling of BMW.

7.2 BIOMEDICAL WASTE MANAGEMENT—DIRECTIVE POLICIES

Biomedical waste disposal and policy are developed on international agreements like the Basel Convention, the Stockholm Convention, and the Minamata Convention. The Basel Convention is a global environmental agreement on hazardous waste. It aims to protect the environment and human health from the harmful consequences of the disposal and handling of waste generated, hazardous waste from hospitals and health centres (Geneva: Basel Convention and United Nations Environment Programme, 2011). The Minamata Convention is an international agreement. It is intended to protect human health and the environment from releases of mercury and mercury compounds. The treaty includes a ban on new mercury mines and limits on the use of mercury in many medical device products, such as blood pressure monitors and thermometers. Due to the unavailability of global regulatory procedures for medical waste, most countries have established their own procedures. WHO reports that uncontrolled and unregulated disposal of high-risk medical waste causes environmental pollution and poses public health risks (Seck, 2012). WHO surveyed biomedical waste management in 24 Western Pacific countries: Japan, China, Australia, New Zealand, Philippines, Malaysia, Vietnam, Cambodia, South Korea, Micronesia, Nauru, and Kiribati. The study was evaluated based on five main areas of biomedical waste: management, policies, training, policy and regulatory frameworks, implemented technologies, and financial resources. All Western Pacific countries except Micronesia, Nauru, and Kiribati have shown satisfactory progress in management, training, and policies related to biomedical waste management. The Republic of Korea and Japan are the only countries that use the best biomedical waste treatment and disposal technology that has been systematically and routinely tested. The remaining countries had no means or no economical means of disposing of biomedical waste. As a result, medical waste management in most Western Pacific countries could be better. The main solution for disposing of biomedical waste is its incineration. The government of India introduced the first biomedical waste regulations in July 1998 under the Ministry of Environment and Forests. The number of incinerators increased rapidly after this (Mattiello et al., 2013). The first standard manual on the safe management of waste from medical activities was published by WHO in 1999 under the name Blue Book.

7.3 BIOMEDICAL WASTE GENERATION AND SEGREGATION IN THE PANDEMIC PERIOD (COVID-19)

Biomedical waste in developing countries is not correctly segregated at the source, increasing exponentially (Nzediegwu & Chang, 2020). According to the Ministry of Environment and Forests (MoEF), India's total biomedical waste generation is 405,702 kg /day, of which only 291,983kg /day is disposed of; the rest of the waste is left untreated and later dumped into the surrounding environment. In a normal situation (non-pandemic), a medical facility generates an average amount of healthcare waste, and the highest rate of generation of healthcare waste occurs in maternity wards and hospitals (Table.7.1). India faced severe consequences during the COVID-19 pandemic, with a huge caseload due to lack of resources and biomedical waste management systems (Anwerand Faizan, 2020).

TABLE 7.1 Average Waste Generation Rates by Different Types of Healthcare Facilities

SOURCES	*TOTAL HEALTHCARE WASTE GENERATION RATE*	*INFECTIOUS HEALTHCARE WASTE GENERATION RATE*
Hospital	2 kg per bed day	0.5 kg per bed day
Clinic	0.02 kg per patient day	0.007 kg per patient day
Maternity centre	5 kg per patient day	3 kg per patient day
Clinical laboratory	0.06 kg per test day	0.02 kg per test day
Basic health unit	0.04 kg per patient day	0.01 kg per patient day

(*Source:* UNEP, 2020)

According to the annual report published by Central Environmental Management Board (CPCB), 2018/2019, BMW production in 2017 was 557 tons/day, of which 517 tons/day were processed. There are currently 198 common biomedical waste management facilities (CBMWFs) approved by the CPCB in India, with another 28 under construction. The COVID-19 pandemic has further unexpectedly increased the amount of BMW coming out of hospitals, laboratories, and quarantine centres. Calculating the exact amount of BMW is very difficult, but some studies show that BMW generation has increased sixfold compared to the pre-pandemic situation (Ma et al., 2020). According to a report submitted by India's CPCB to the National Green Tribunal (NGT) on June 17, 2020, 101 tons of biomedical waste related to COVID-19 and more than 601 tons of other biomedical waste are being produced. In the pre-pandemic era, hospitals produced an average of $500-750$ g BMW per bed per day, which now has increased to $2.5-4.5\,\text{kg}$. These data recommend the segregation of domestic waste generated from BMW to reduce the load on incinerators handling BMW.

7.4 STEPS INVOLVED IN COVID-19–ASSOCIATED BIOMEDICAL WASTE MANAGEMENT

7.4.1 Step I—Segregation

Waste segregation should be done at the point of generation to avoid mixing with municipal waste. All BMW waste generated during COVID-19 pandemic is segregated into various colour-coded bags, containers, or boxes (refer to Chapters 6 and 8 for details regarding segregation).

7.4.2 Step II—Packaging

Before packaging the waste, cleaning of surroundings and smooth surfaces requires cleaning the surface with water and cleanser followed by application of sanitizer (0.1% sodium hypochlorite or 72–92 % ethanol). The minimum required contact time is 60 seconds for ethanol, chlorine-based materials, and H_2O_2 (hydrogen peroxide) more than 0.49% with purifier residues requiring clean water cleaning. All BMW should be collected and segregated onsite in yellow/red bags, blue cardboard, and white puncture-proof vessels (Chand et al., 2021) (refer to Chapters 6 and 8 for details regarding packaging).

7.4.3 Step III—Transportation

Generated BMW should not be stored for more than 24 hours. The collected waste material should be stowed in well-aired designated storage areas and carried to waste treatment facilities for additional disposal. This segregated waste should be conveyed in a designated closed vehicle with a global locating system tracker to a common biomedical waste disposal facility for final disposal. After every trip, these vehicles should be sanitized with 1% hypochlorite (Chand et al., 2021) (refer to Chapters 6 and 8 for details regarding packaging).

7.5 COVID-19–ASSOCIATED BIOMEDICAL WASTE MANAGEMENT—TREATMENT STRATEGIES

Following are the different methods used while disposing of biomedical waste, such as chemical processes, thermal processes, mechanical processes, irradiation processes, and biological processes.

7.5.1 Chemical Processes

COVID-19–associated biomedical waste is initially treated with a chemical disinfection technique before it is mechanically shredded. Chemical disinfectants are applied due to their properties: effectiveness at low concentrations, rapid action, stable performance, and broad sterilization spectrum. Such chemicals include sodium hypochlorite, dissolved chlorine dioxide, peracetic acid, hydrogen peroxide, dry inorganic chemicals, and ozone. Most chemical processes require large amounts of water and neutralizing agents (Emmanuel et al., 2001).

7.5.2 Thermal Processes

Low-heat systems: These include systems operating between $93°C$ and $177°C$. Examples include microwaves and autoclaves (Emmanuel et al., 2001). Autoclaves use steam under pressure as a method for sterilization, which facilities disinfect types of equipment supplied contaminated with infectious biohazardous agents, surgical instruments, and supplies. Equipment inside the autoclave chamber is heated at temperatures ranging from $121°C$ to $132°C$ $(250-270°F)$ (Lipman & Leary, 2015). Hazardous waste and chemicals cannot be autoclaved, as they release toxic emissions (Emmanuel et al., 2001). Microwaves use moist heat and steam to disinfect. All infectious waste, including human, laboratory, and soft waste, is sterilized in a microwave before discarding. The advantage of using microwaves for biomedical waste disposal is that they have minimum emissions.

High-heat systems: These include systems operating at temperatures ranging from $550^{\circ}C$ to $8500^{\circ}C$. This includes oxidation, plasma pyrolysis, induction-based pyrolysis, and lase-based pyrolysis. During the pyrolysis process inside the pyrolysis chamber, the thermal breakdown of the organic solid and liquid waste vaporizes at high temperatures in an inert atmosphere $(590°C)$, leaving behind inert ash and fragments. The next step is the combustion of the vapours in a chamber at a temperature of $980°C-1090°C$, and clean exhaust steam is later released (Nema & Ganeshprasad, 2002).

Incineration: This method of extraordinary temperature combustion is used from $800°C$ to $1200°C$. It results in burning up to 90% of carbon-based matter and complete killing of the pathogen. Currently, most COVID BMW is incinerated at a temperature of more than $1100°C$. Later, the residual mass is re-incinerated if required.

Alternative thermal techniques: Two types of alternative thermal technology are available and are practiced to deal with COVID-19 waste: (1) the high-temperature pyrolysis technique and (2) the medium-temperature micro-wave technique. Pyrolysis is a technologically more advanced technique than incineration. It usually operates in the temperature range of $540-830$ °C with techniques comprising pyrolysis-oxidation, plasma pyrolysis, induction-based pyrolysis, and laser-based pyrolysis (Datta et al., 2018). Because of the rapid spread potential of SARS-CoV-2, using plasma energy for quick decomposition of COVID waste is recommended over the usual laser/gaseous combustion (Wang et al., 2020).

7.5.3 Mechanical Processes

These processes are used to modify the physical form or properties of waste to facilitate its handling or to treat it in combination with other treatment steps. Two fundamental processes are the following:

- Reducing the volume of the waste by a process called compaction.
- Destruction of plastic and paper waste by shredder; this process (known as shredding) prevents reuse of materials.

7.5.4 Irradiation Processes

Ionizing radiation is helpful in BMW management, as it damages the DNA, proteins, and enzymes of infectious particles. Electron beam technology, with the production of ionizing radiation, is used at high speed to strike the target. Infectious waste includes human excrement, laboratory waste, ward waste, and blades. This process does not produce toxic emissions and no liquid effluent or ionizing radiation. The machine has low operational cost and is fully automated (Emmanuel et al., 2001).

7.5.5 Biological Processes

This method includes an emerging "bio-converter" system to dispose of bio-medical waste. During this process, the medical waste is first decontaminated with a solution of enzymes. The resulting sludge is put through an extruder to remove sewage disposal, and the remaining solid waste is discarded in a landfill. Biodegradable plastics and biomedical implants are examples of environment-friendly biomedical waste disposal (Roy & Choudhury, 2022). Such plastics are built to undergo biological degradation with microbial extracellular enzymes. Further research is required to manufacture biodegradable plastics (Datta et al., 2018).

7.6 OCCUPATIONAL SAFETY AND HEALTH

Waste generated in healthcare facilities can threaten the lives of workers, patients, and facility personnel if not properly handled or disposed of (Aluko et al., 2016). The potential for occupational infections from medical waste in developing countries is much higher than in developed countries. In some medical centres, medical waste is disposed of together with general waste, which can lead to increased rates of communicable and non-communicable diseases (Polan et al., 2013). Occupational exposure to medical waste can be prevented by following standard procedures for waste sorting, treatment, and disposal (Polan et al., 2013). Common precautions include washing hands and wearing protective equipment, including face shields, boots, gloves, aprons, and personal protective equipment. Apart from precautions when handling waste, vaccination of workers against preventable occupational infections should be included. Implementation of safety regulations varies by country and by medical facility. Some centres have deplorable safety measures, which can cause serious health problems for those who handle medical waste.

7.7 POLICY AND REGULATORY FRAMEWORK

Rules and regulations for medical waste disposal are in place to avoid illegal and improper disposal of generated waste. Illegal dumping sites exist on the outskirts of many cities, causing several health problems. To avoid this problem, the Ministry of Environment and Forests established regulations for biomedical waste in 1998 under the Environmental Protection Act. In accordance with these regulations, necessary steps must be taken by those in higher positions and with authority over work facilities to ensure the proper and safe disposal of waste generated in healthcare facilities. 2016 the government of India (GOI) reviewed the Regulations on Disposal of Biomedical Medical Waste (1998). This law defines the obligations of users and operators, and the obligations of users include disposing of the waste produced without harming the environment or human health. Various state governments have also implemented solid waste management regulations under the Biomedical Waste Management Regulations 2016 and the Central Discharge Control Board. Some workers highlighted the requirement for properly monitoring environmental protection regulations and regulations (Nwachukwu et al., 2013).

7.8 SAFE HANDLING OF COVID-19–ASSOCIATED BIOMEDICAL WASTE

Safe disposal of biomedical waste is not the only concern; it also includes the safety of workers handling the waste. Waste treatment related to biomedical waste includes the entire process of waste generation, sorting, grouping, storage, transport, treatment, and final disposal. According to the Biomedical Waste Management Regulations (2016), it is up to each individual to ensure that all necessary measures are taken to prevent adverse effects on the environment and human health during biomedical waste disposal. It is the duty of the manager of the institution.

The following are some important points to remember about safe handling of biomedical waste:

- Supervisors' instructions on how to dispose of waste must be carefully followed.
- Ask your trainer about how to dispose of different types of waste and what to do if you come in contact with a hypodermic needle or need personal protective equipment.
- Wear a PPE kit and steel-toed boots to protect yourself when handling hazardous waste. Gloves should be worn to protect the hands from debris, and cover the arms and the rest of the skin surface to prevent unnecessary injury.
- Avoid direct contact with medical waste, especially red bags, with your bare hands, feet, or skin. Always cover all kinds of cuts and scrapes on duty.
- In the event of a spill, special equipment such as respirators, face shields, face masks, and boot swabs should be worn to protect against splashes.
- Never touch glass shards or sharp objects directly with an uncovered hand.

REFERENCES

Aluko, O. O., Adebayo, A. E., Adebisi, T. F., Ewegbemi, M. K., Abidoye, A. T., & Popoola, B. F. (2016). Knowledge, attitudes, and perceptions of occupational hazards and safety practices in Nigerian healthcare workers. *BMC Research Notes*, *9*(1), 1–14.

Chand, S., Shastry, C. S., Hiremath, S., Joel, J. J., Krishnabhat, C. H., & Mateti, U. V. (2021). Updates on biomedical waste management during COVID-19: The Indian scenario. *Clinical Epidemiology and Global Health*, *11*, 100715.

Choudhury, M., Sahoo, S., Samanta, P., Tiwari, A., Tiwari, A., Chadha, U., & Chakravorty, A. (2022). COVID-19: An accelerator for global plastic consumption and its implications. *Journal of Environmental and Public Health*, *2022*.

Datta, P., Mohi, G., & Chander, J. (2018). Biomedical waste management in India: Critical appraisal. *Journal of Laboratory Physicians*, *10*(1), 006–014.

Emmanuel, J., Puccia, C. J., & Spurgin, R. A. (2001). *Non-incineration medical waste treatment technologies*. Health Care Without Harm.

Karliner, J., Slotterback, S., Boyd, R., Ashby, B., Steele, K., & Wang, J. (2020). Health care's climate footprint: The health sector contribution and opportunities for action. *European Journal of Public Health*, *30*(Supplement_5), ckaa165–843.

Lipman, N. S., & Leary, S. L. (2015). Design and management of research facilities. In *Laboratory animal medicine* (pp. 1543–1597). Academic Press.

Ma, Y., Lin, X., Wu, A., Huang, Q., Li, X., & Yan, J. (2020). Suggested guidelines for emergency treatment of medical waste during COVID-19: Chinese experience. *Waste Disposal & Sustainable Energy*, *2*, 81–84.

Mattiello, A., Chiodini, P., Bianco, E., Forgione, N., Flammia, I., Gallo, C., . . . & Panico, S. (2013). Health effects associated with the disposal of solid waste in landfills and incinerators in populations living in surrounding areas: A systematic review. *International Journal of Public Health*, *58*, 725–735.

Minoglou, M., Gerassimidou, S., & Komilis, D. (2017). Healthcare waste generation worldwide and its dependence on socio-economic and environmental factors. *Sustainability*, *9*(2), 220.

Nema, S. K., & Ganeshprasad, K. S. (2002). Plasma pyrolysis of medical waste. *Current Science*, 271–278.

Nwachukwu, N. C., Orji, F. A., & Ugbogu, O. C. (2013). Health care waste management–public health benefits, and the need for effective environmental regulatory surveillance in federal Republic of Nigeria. *Current Topics in Public Health*, *2*, 149–178.

Nzediegwu, C., & Chang, S. X. (2020). Improper solid waste management increases potential for COVID-19 spread in developing countries. *Resources, Conservation, and Recycling*, *161*, 104947.

Peng, J., Wu, X., Wang, R., Li, C., Zhang, Q., & Wei, D. (2020). Medical waste management practice during the 2019–2020 novel coronavirus pandemic: Experience in a general hospital. *American Journal of Infection Control*, *48*(8), 918–921.

Polan, M. A. A., Al Noman, N., Jan, C. M., Hasan, M. R., & Saito, T. (2013). Practice and knowledge of health personnel on impact of medical wastes in Upazilla Health Complexes under Dhaka Division in Bangladesh. *City Dental College Journal*, *10*(1), 1–4.

Roy, P., & Choudhury, M. (2022). Bioeconomy and green plastic production. *Encyclopedia of Green Materials*, 1–7.

Seck, S. L. (2012). Home state regulation of environmental human rights harms as transnational private regulatory governance. *German Law Journal*, *13*(12), 1363–1385.

Secretariat of the Basel Convention. (2011). *Technical guidelines on environmentally sound management of wastes consisting of elemental mercury and wastes containing or contaminated with Mercury 31 October, 2011*. Basel Convention and United Nations Environment Programme.

Song, Y., Ye, J., Liu, Y., & Zhong, Y. (2021). *Estimation of solid medical waste production and environmental impact analysis in the context of COVID-19: A case study of Hubei province in China*.

Tenglikar, P. V., Kumar, G. A., Kapate, R., Reddy, S., & Vijayanath, V. (2012). Knowledge attitude and practices of health care waste management amongst staff of nursing homes of Gulbarga city. *Journal of Pharmaceutical and Biomedical Sciences*, *19*(12), 1–3.

Wang, J., Shen, J., Ye, D., Yan, X., Zhang, Y., Yang, W., . . . & Pan, L. (2020). Disinfection technology of hospital wastes and wastewater: Suggestions for disinfection strategy during coronavirus Disease 2019 (COVID-19) pandemic in China. *Environmental Pollution*, *262*, 114665.

8 Biomedical Waste Management

Legal and Regulatory Framework and Remedial Strategies

Nilofer Hussaini, Sunitha Abhay Jain, Tajwar Hussaini, Daisy Alexander, Sunil John, and Bidisha Sarkar

8.1 INTRODUCTION

Bio-medical waste management (BMW) has occupied the centre stage in discussion and deliberation amongst legislators, environmentalists, policy-makers, and stakeholders worldwide. After the onset of COVID, the quantity of bio-medical waste in hospitals, health care centres, and household units has increased considerably. The volume of waste mainly includes personal protective gear such as hand gloves, face masks and shields, white

DOI: 10.1201/9781003499695-8

gowns, rubber boots, and hand sanitizers and other equipment such as plastic containers, syringes, bandages, tissues, and test kits that have a high contamination rate. Millions of people have been infected and have lost their lives due to the pandemic. As of 1 October 2021, WHO reported that there had been 233,503,524 confirmed cases, including 4,777,503 deaths. As of 28 September 2021, 6,143,369,655 vaccine doses had been administered (WHO, 2021b). The unprecedented rise in the number of cases and deaths and consequent generation of waste has put a lot of pressure on the healthcare services and waste management infrastructure. The rate at which medical waste is generated has increased considerably due to the diagnosis and treatment of COVID-19. In 2020, it was reported that there was a 23% hike in the generation of medical waste in China alone (Asian Development Bank, 2020). India recorded an increase of 250 tonnes of medical waste in the same year (CPCB, 2021). The World Health Organization (WHO, 2021) estimated that more than 15 billion injections were used yearly, but all were not safely disposed of. In October 2020, UNICEF announced that it would stockpile 520 million syringes worldwide to prepare for the COVID-19 vaccination, with a target of 1 billion syringes in 2021 (UNICEF, 2020). Syringes are not the only item contributing to the increase in medical waste in 2020. Face masks, medical kits, gloves, and other similar items are also significant hazardous contributors (Choudhury et al., 2022). Table 8.1 shows the increased amount of BMW produced from hospital care facilities during the pandemic in selected cities of the world, Table 8.2 depicts average waste generated at various sources, and Table 8.3 shows comparative data of total and hazardous waste generated in various countries.

TABLE 8.1 Increased BMW due to COVID-19

CITIES	*POPULATION*	*MEDICAL WASTE GENERATED BEFORE COVID (TONNES/DAY)*	*ADDITIONAL MEDICAL WASTE DURING COVID (TONNES/DAY)*	*PERCENTAGE OF RISE IN WASTE DURING COVID*
Manila	14 million	47	280	496
Jakarta	10.6 million	35	212	506
Bangkok	10.5 million	35	210	500
Hanoi	8 million	27	160	493
Kuala Lumpur	7.7 million	26	154	492

(*Source:* UNEP, 2020)

TABLE 8.2 Average Waste Generated at Various Stages

HEALTH FACILITY	*TOTAL WASTE GENERATED*	*INFECTIOUS WASTE GENERATED*
Hospitals	2 kgs/patient/day	0.5 kgs/patient/day
Clinics	0.02 kgs/patient/day	0.007 kgs/patient/day
Maternity centres	5 kgs/patient/day	3 kgs/patient/day
Clinical laboratories	0.06 kgs/patient/day	0.02 kgs/patient/day
Basic healthcare units	0.04 kgs/patient/day	0.01 kgs/patient/day

(*Source:* WHO, 2014)

TABLE 8.3 Total and Hazardous Waste Generated in Selected Countries

COUNTRIES/FACILITIES	*TOTAL HEALTHCARE WASTE GENERATED (KG/BED/DAY)*	*HAZARDOUS WASTE GENERATED (KG/PATIENT/DAY)*
Pakistan		
Hospitals	2.07	
Consulting clinics and dispensaries	0.1	0.063
Basic healthcare units	0.04	0.03
Nursing homes	0.3	
Maternity homes	4.1	2.9
Tanzania		
Hospitals	0.14	0.08
Healthcare centres	0.01	0.007
Clinics and dispensaries	0.06	0.03
South Africa		
National hospitals		1.24
Provincial hospitals		1.53
Regional hospitals		1.05
District hospitals		0.65
Specialized hospitals		0.17

(*Source:* WHO, 2014)

8.2 BIO-MEDICAL WASTE MANAGEMENT: LEGAL AND REGULATORY FRAMEWORK

8.2.1 International Perspective

In order to address the issue of bio-medical waste around the world, several international conventions and agreements have been agreed upon and signed by countries to protect health and the environment and to take steps for safe disposal of waste. These international agreements and conventions can be considered for formulation of waste-management strategies, policies, and legislation. Some of the important international conventions are discussed subsequently.

8.2.1.1 Basel Convention on the Control of Trans-Boundary Movement of Hazardous Waste and their Disposal, 1992 (Basel Convention, 1992)

It is one of the most important international environment treaties dealing with waste that is hazardous in nature. The Convention was signed by 170 member nations, and its objective is to protect the environment and human health from ill effects of production, transportation, and disposal of waste which is hazardous in nature. It is pertinent to follow the principle of "prior informed consent" where there is movement of waste which is hazardous across boundaries. All signatories are required to initiate suitable municipal laws to intercept and penalize illegal movement of waste of a hazardous nature. An obligation is imposed on the parties to the convention to manage and dispose of high-risk and other wastes in an environmental friendly manner. Signatories are expected to minimize the generation of waste in their respective countries to avoid transportation of huge quantities of waste across borders. The Basel Convention also classifies hazardous wastes into different categories, such as Y1, which refers to clinical wastes generated at hospital facilities and medical care units. Further, the Y3 category includes unwanted and expired drugs and medicines and associated wastes. Under Annexure III, UN Class Code H6.2, of the convention, a list of characteristics which are hazardous is given. Further, an infectious substance has been defined as a substance that contains micro-organisms or their toxins which can cause disease in animals as well as humans. The Convention Secretariat also issued comprehensive guidelines for managing bio-medical waste to ensure a sustainable environment (Prüss et al., 1999). Two major restrictions are given in the Basel Convention regarding waste movements.

The first restriction imposes certain conditions for the export of waste: it can occur only under the certain circumstances such as when the country does not have adequate facilities for disposal or recycling in an environmentally friendly manner or when the waste can be used as raw material in the importing country. The second restriction relates to trans-boundary transportation of waste between parties and non-parties on the basis of a separate agreement.

8.2.1.2 Convention on the Import into Africa and the Control of Trans-Boundary Movement and Management of Hazardous Wastes within Africa, Bamako, 1998

It was formed as a response to the failure of the Basel Convention to prohibit the import of waste hazardous to Africa. This treaty was negotiated in January 1991 amongst 12 nations belonging to the Organization of African Unity, which came into force in the year 1998.

8.2.1.3 Convention on Persistent Organic Pollutants (POPs), Stockholm 2004 (United Nations Treaty Collection, 2001)

This convention came into force on 17 May 2004 in Stockholm, Sweden. This convention mainly focuses on eliminating and reducing the release of POPs in the atmosphere for a long time, which accumulate in the tissue of living organisms and can prove to be toxic. The convention also deals with tackling additional chemicals identified as impermissible hazardous materials. The importance of the convention is that it paved the way for the future generation, which would be free of dangerous POPs and reduce reliance on toxic chemicals. Signatories to this convention must take steps to reduce or eliminate the release of harmful chemicals produced during incineration or other high-temperature treatments by using standardized techniques and practices for a sustainable environment. The convention contains guidelines that prescribe technologies such as advanced steam sterilization, hot-air disinfection treatment, microwave techniques, alkaline hydrolysis, and biological techniques to reduce the release of harmful chemicals into the atmosphere (WHO, 2014).

8.2.2 Indian Perspective

Before the Bio-Medical Waste (BMW) Management Rules, 1998 (Ministry of Environment and Forests, 1998), there was no proper system, and bio-medical waste management was inadequate. Scavengers were ones who sorted out the waste, and there was no mechanism to protect and guard them against its ill effects (Salkin, 2004). This practice endangered their health and the environment, as they sorted the waste with bare hands, and no protective gear was used. There was also no proper method by which waste could be recycled, and rampant reuse of improper sterilized syringes was common. In July 1998, the Ministry of Forest and Environment issued the Bio-Medical Waste Management Rules. Various changes were made to these rules in 2000, 2003, and 2011. In March 2016, the Ministry of Environment, Forest and Climate amended the Bio-Medical Waste Management Rules, increasing the scope.

8.2.2.1 Salient Features of Bio-Medical Waste Management Rules, 2016

1. Under the Bio-Medical Waste Management Rules, 2016, the Central Pollution Control Board (CPCB) and the State Pollution Control Committees (SPCCs) are entrusted to withdraw the authorization of healthcare institutions and hospital facilities that do not comply with the rules. The hospital officials, staff, and attendants must follow directives relating to the waste generated at the source. Waste handlers such as *safai karmacharis*, attendants, and sanitation staff must be well trained to handle bio-medical waste. The medical, dental, and paramedical staff should know the guidelines for handling and managing bio-medical waste. The World Health Organization and the National AIDS Organization Control have prescribed that all health workers in India should be trained and immunized against diseases.
2. Waste from vaccination, surgical, and blood donation camps is included under the Bio-Medical Waste Management Rules. Further, the rule also specified the duties of occupiers and operators. Healthcare facilities with more than 1000 beds must obtain authorization.
3. The Bio-Medical Waste Management Rules, 2016, categorized waste into four categories based on treatment and disposal methods.
4. Containers and bags used for the collection and storage of waste should be clearly marked with the biohazard and cytotoxic hazard symbols. A barcode system for bio-medical waste sent for treatment or disposal has been set up.
5. In consensus with World Health Organization guidelines, the Indian Bio-Medical Waste Management Rules included the compulsory pretreatment (through disinfection and sterilization on site) of laboratory waste, microbiological waste, blood samples, and blood bags.

6. Stringent high standards must be followed regarding pollutants emitted in the environment from incinerators. In case of any major accidents or fire accidents occurring while handling bio-medical waste, proper procedures have been laid down in the prescribed format to seek remedial action.
7. Hospitals or healthcare centres prohibit on-site treatment of bio-medical waste. The rules also prescribe setting up a common bio-medical waste management treatment facility within 75 kilometres. The common bio-medical treatment and disposal facility operators should ensure the timely collection of bio-medical waste from the healthcare facility and assist the healthcare facility in conducting training (Ministry of Environment, Forests and Climate Change, 2016). Table 8.4 deals with the various schedules as envisaged under the Bio-Medical Waste Management Rules of 1998 and 2016. Table 8.5 deals with various forms under the 2016 rules used for different purposes, such as accident reporting and renewal authorisation, amongst others.

TABLE 8.4 Schedules Prescribed under Bio-Medical Waste Management Rules, 1998 and 2016

SCHEDULE	*1998*	*2016*
Schedule 1	Waste categories.	Colour coding, waste type, treatment, and disposal.
Schedule 2	Waste type, colour coding, category of waste, treatment options.	Standard for treatment and management of disposal of biomedical waste (autoclaving/microwaving/deep burial, dry heat sterilization/chemical disinfection).
Schedule 3	Labels of biomedical waste categories/bags.	Prescribed authority list and duties.
Schedule 4	Labels for transport of biomedical waste.	Container/bag: Part A label. Transport of container/bag: Part B label.
Schedule 5	Treatment standards, management of disposal of biomedical waste.	Added to schedule 2.
Schedule 6	List of prescribed authorities and duties.	Added to schedule 3.

(*Source:* Datta et al., 2018)

TABLE 8.5 Various Forms in the Bio-Medical Waste Management Rules, 2016

FORMS	*USE OF FORMS*
F1	Accident reporting.
F2	Authorization/renewal application.
F3	Generation, collection, storage, transport, treatment, disposal authorization.
F4	Yearly report.
F5	Appeal application against the order passed.

(*Source:* Datta et al., 2018)

8.2.2.2 Bio-Medical Waste Management (Amendment) Rules, 2018

In 2018, the Ministry of Environment, Forest and Climate Change brought about amendments to these rules. According to these amended rules, instead of 10% sodium hypochlorite, 1% to 2% sodium hypochlorite with 30% residual chlorine should be used for bio-medical waste treatment. The important aspects of the rules were:

1. To completely phase out chlorinated plastic items such as bags and gloves from bio-medical waste.
2. To compulsorily publish annual reports on the websites of medical institutions.
3. To establish global positioning and the barcoding system by the operators to handle bio-medical waste framed by the Central Pollution Control Board guidelines.
4. To send reports to the Central Pollution Control Board by State Pollution Control Boards after compiling, reviewing, and analysing the information received by the operators.

8.3 BIO-MEDICAL WASTE MANAGEMENT REMEDIAL MEASURES IN SELECT COUNTRIES

Actions involving the implementation of effective healthcare waste management programs require both a short-term and long-term approach. They require multi-sectorial collaboration and interaction at all levels. For effective implementation, waste management policies must be generated globally and integrated locally for best management practices. Different countries have their own pre-existing regulations for waste management. The level of implementation of regulations differs from country to country depending upon various factors such as divergent economic conditions, population, and so on. The bio-medical waste management remedial mechanisms of different countries are discussed in the following.

8.3.1 United Kingdom

It has been observed that National Healthcare Services (NHS), Cornwall, faces major waste management challenges due to infrastructural and organizational structure limitations. Certain barriers, such as public perceptions and staff habits, have also been noticed. Considering these issues, an overall waste management mechanism has been designed in which waste audits were implemented to check redundant equipment, bulky waste, clinical bags, and special waste from different medical sites. The NHS attempted to overcome the gap and effectively progress between waste management and minimization. The NHS has undertaken certain initiatives to improve the overall organizational infrastructure and enhance localized control. A strategic partnership between and within sites has been recommended to the NHS, along with collaboration with the local community. Staff training and awareness programs have been considered to minimize the waste at the source, executing several short-, medium-, and long-term solutions. A study estimated that these solutions could potentially lessen the quantity of disposal by 20–30% (approx.) and costs by approximately 25–35% (Tudor et al., 2005).

8.3.2 Indonesia

The operation of healthcare bio-medical waste management in Indonesia is segregated into two categories, on-site and off-site (Figure 8.1). It has been decided that for COVID-19 waste, specific precautions need to be taken which may require additional operations for both on-site and off-site locations. The Indonesian government follows waste management remedial mechanisms as given subsequently.

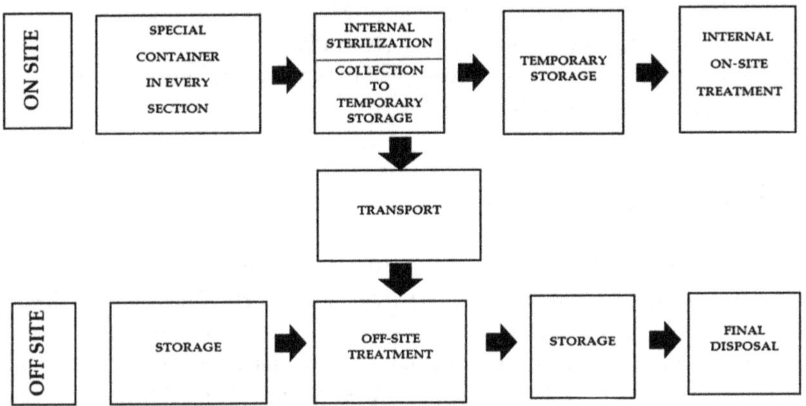

FIGURE 8.1 Onsite and offsite flow of management of COVID-19 waste.

Source: Tsukiji et al., 2020

1. Waste storage should be carried out in sealed packages but not more than 2 days post-production.
2. Waste should be burned with incineration temperature at least 800°C.
3. Combustion residue should be appropriately packed in a specific colour-coded container. They should be properly labelled as hazardous toxic waste. After labelling, they should be stored in a specific storage site.
4. A manager should be allotted to handle toxic and hazardous waste, and all the containers or residue should be transported to this manager for further treatment.
5. Waste such as masks, gloves, PPE, and others should be packed in a container which should clearly be labelled as "Infectious Waste".
6. Collections should be carried out by the concerned Department of Environmental Hygiene and Health officers. Later, waste is sent to the respective collection centres before transporting it for toxic and hazardous waste processing.

A few initiatives were undertaken by the Indonesian government to manage household waste and channel it properly during COVID-19:

1. Encourage households to reduce COVID-19–related waste by adopting reusable products that can be used further after washing.

2. Educate households with proper trashing mechanisms, indicating the tearing and cutting of disposable PPE.
3. Local governments were requested to prepare drop boxes and trash in public places (UNEP, 2020)

8.3.3 Kenya

The Environment Management and Coordination Regulation (2006) in Kenya regulates health care and bio-medical waste management. The authority developed two policies for effective health care waste management: the National Policy on Injection Safety and Medical Waste Management, 2007 and the National Infection Prevention and Control Guidelines for Healthcare Services, 2010. In 2020, the Safety Management and Disposal of Safety Products in Prevention of Spread of COVID-19 was developed. The operation process is as follows:

1. A double-chamber incinerator should be placed for infectious waste, and post-incinerated ashes should be disposed of in an ash pit.
2. Infectious waste coming out of health centres and dispensaries should be burned in oil drum incinerators. Guidelines also suggest that solid waste disposal mechanisms should be such that they are not hazardous to the environment.
3. For general healthcare waste, regular community disposal sites should be identified.
4. For a basic incineration process, locally available materials should be used, such as bricks, oil drums, and concrete blocks (UNEP, 2020).

8.3.4 Sri Lanka

The Sri Lankan government framed interim guidelines for bio-medical waste management by households under a COVID-19 self-quarantine protocol. The interim guidelines were issued in April 2020 and were proposed in line with the present standard, regulation, and management policy. However, provision was made to accommodate the specific emergency situation to manage waste by local Sri-Lankan authorities. Health care waste management practices in Sri Lanka are presented in Figure 8.2.

<table>
<tr><th>Waste Management Flow</th><th>Organic Waste</th><th>Non-Biodegradable Waste</th><th>Special Waste</th></tr>
<tr><td>Treatment for COVID-19 waste</td><td>Not to be placed into compost facilities or allowed to be scavenged by any person or animal</td><td>Incinerate if a facility available</td><td>Mandatory thermal treatment (i.e., incineration) for special waste; if not available, waste should be handed over to accredited clinical waste handler for safe treatment through combustion</td></tr>
<tr><td>Disposal (on-site)</td><td>Households with adequate space are recommended to construct a waste disposal pit to dispose all organic waste on-site: minimum 2 ft deep secured with bunds around the pit. Waste is to be disinfected prior to disposing in the pit</td><td>Consider on-site disposal due to unavailability or difficulty of providing normal waste collection service. Excavate a pit (2 × 2 × 2 ft) on ground & place waste bags in the pit. Waste is to be disinfected prior to disposing in the pit. Waste should be covered by 6-inch-thick soil layer</td><td>N/A</td></tr>
<tr><td>Disposal (off-site)</td><td colspan="2">Sanitary landfill if available. Emergency land disposal 8 ft deep; must not reach underground water level. Prevent rainwater entering by soil ridge and furrows. Protected from the reach of people and animals. Waste is to be disinfected prior to disposal. Disposed waste should be covered by soil</td><td>N/A</td></tr>
</table>

TABLE 8.6 Operation based on waste category.

Source: Tsukiji et al., 2020

8.4 BIO-MEDICAL WASTE MANAGEMENT: ISSUES AND CHALLENGES

Countries worldwide are facing various issues and challenges regarding bio-medical waste management. Many developing countries, such as Bangladesh, India, Malaysia, the Philippines, Vietnam, Cambodia, and Thailand, have poor waste management systems (Sangkham, 2020). Developing countries face various challenges due to inadequate and inappropriate handling of waste. Low-income countries need to deal with the increased amount of biomedical waste generation, as they have prohibited the segregation and reprocessing of waste to combat COVID-19. A common practice amongst low-income countries is mixing medical waste with municipal waste. One more concern is that, in low-income countries, bio-medical waste is not segregated into hazardous and non-hazardous categories (WHO, 2018). Contamination can also result from bio-medical waste such as blood, fluids, swabs, tissues, and organs. Regulation of bio-medical waste management in developing countries becomes difficult due to weak and inadequate regulations. Improper management of bio-medical waste can cause many diseases like AIDS; meningitis; and skin, eye, intestinal, and respiratory infections. Manual sorting of infectious waste and large-scale scavenging at waste dumps and healthcare establishments have resulted in workers' poor health. The toxic chemicals and radioactive waste from bio-medical waste can cause air, water, and land pollution. Disposal of bio-medical waste involves burning or incineration, which releases toxic and harmful gases into the atmosphere, resulting in air pollution and a threat to public health. Further, it has led to a depletion of the ozone layer and has contributed to the greenhouse effect. Improper disposal of bio-medical waste and dumping in landfills can contaminate the surface and groundwater. Due to various chemicals in this waste, they may get mixed with the soil and change its composition, which may lower its quality. Nearly 1.6 million tonnes of plastic was generated due to the use of masks, PPE kits, sanitizers, gloves, and aprons, which were not discarded properly during the pandemic, resulting in the accumulation of plastics along the coastlines and sea beds, threatening marine life. The rampant re-use of disposable needles and syringes is a serious cause of concern in countries such as African, Central Asian, and Eastern European countries (Zafar, 2019). Many different biocidal agents, soaps, and detergents are used to wash the contaminated material used in treating COVID-19 patients. This, in turn, is also a potential threat to water bodies.

Bio-medical waste management is still in its initial stages and needs further development. Sound management of waste, such as municipal solid waste, health care waste, and e-waste, is crucial for protecting the environment and health. In most developing countries, there is less awareness, ineffective implementation of laws, minimum participation of stakeholders, and lack of resources such as technical and financial expertise about bio-medical waste management systems. Some additional challenges include insufficient training and education regarding bio-medical waste segregation and clearance. Other areas of concern include improper storage disposal, lack of awareness, inefficient treatment procedures, and lack of proper technology and expertise. It is important to put in place safe burial practices and cremation of dead COVID-19 patients. Countries should take a lot of precautions while burying dead patients to prevent infection and transmission of the deadly virus. Many countries are facing the challenge of a workforce shortage for waste collection; hence, there is a disruption in waste collection services. It is quite challenging for countries to handle enormous amounts of waste and ensure safe management from the collection point to recycling and treatment facilities.

REFERENCES

Asian Development Bank. (2020). *Managing infectious medical waste during the COVID-19 pandemic*. Asian Development Bank. https://events.development.asia/materials/20200405/managing-infectious-medical-waste-during-covid-19-pandemic

Bamako Convention. (1991). *Bamako convention on the ban of the import into Africa and the control of transboundary movement and management of hazardous wastes within Africa*. Lex Mercatoria.

Basel Convention. (1992). *Basel convention on the control of transboundary movements of hazardous wastes and their disposal*. World Health Organization.

Central Pollution Control Board. (2016). *Guidelines for management of healthcare waste as per biomedical waste management rules 2016*. Government of India, Ministry of Environment, Forest and Climate Change, Directorate General of Health Services Ministry of Health & Family Welfare.

CPCB. (2021). *Generation of COVID19 related biomedical waste in States/UTs*. Central Pollution Control Board, Ministry of Environment, Forest and Climate Change, Government of India. https://cpcb.nic.in/uploads/Projects/Bio-Medical-Waste/COVID19_Waste_Management_status_Jan_May_2021.pdf

Choudhury, M., Sahoo, S., Samanta, P., Tiwari, A., Chadha, U., Bhardwaj, P., Nalluri, A.,Eticha, T.K., & Chakravorty, A. (2022). COVID-19: An accelerator for global plastic consumption and its implications. *Journal of Environmental and Public Health, 2022*. https://doi.org/10.1155/2022/1066350

Datta, P., Mohi, G. K., & Chander, J. (2018). Biomedical waste management in India: Critical appraisal. *Journal of Laboratory Physicians*, *10*(1), 6–14.

Ministry of Environment and Forests. (1998). *Bio-medical waste (Management & Handling) rules, 1998*. Ministry of Environment and Forests.

Ministry of Environment, Forests and Climate Change. (2016). *Bio-medical waste management rules 2016*. Government of India, Ministry of Environment, Forests and Climate Change.

Prüss, A., Giroult, E., & Rushbrook, P. (1999). *Safe management of wastes from health care activities*. World Health Organization. https://apps.who.int/iris/bitstream/handle/10665/42175/9241545259.pdf

Salkin, I. F. (2004). *Review of health impacts from microbiological hazards in health-care wastes.* World Health Organization.

Sangkham, S. (2020, September 30). Face mask and medical waste disposal during the novel COVID-19 pandemic in Asia. *Case Studies in Chemical and Environmental Engineering*, *2*, 1–2. https://doi.org/10.1016/j.cscee.2020.100052

Tsukiji, M, Gamaralalage, P.J.D., Pratomo, I.S.Y, Onogawa, K., Alverson, K., Honda, S., Ternald, D., Dilley, M., Fujioka, J., Condrorini, D. (2020). *Waste management during the COVID-19 pandemic from response to recovery*. United Nations Environment Programme.

Tudor, T., Noonan, C., & Jenkin, L. (2005). Healthcare waste management: A case study from the national health service in Cornwall, United Kingdom. *Waste Management*, *25*(6), 606–615.

UNEP, (2020). *BASEL: waste management an essential public service in the fight to beat COVID-19*. The United Nations Environment Programme (UNEP) and the Basel Convention.

UNICEF. (2020, October). *UNICEF to stockpile over half a billion syringes by year end, as part of efforts to prepare for eventual COVID-19 vaccinations*. UNICEF. https://www.unicef.org/press-releases/unicef-stockpile-over-half-billion-syringes-year-end-part-efforts-prepare-eventual

United Nations Treaty Collection. (2001, May). *Stockholm convention on persistent organic pollutants*. United Nations Treaty Collection. https://treaties.un.org/Pages/ViewDetails.aspx?src=IND&mtdsg_no=XXVII-15&chapter=27&clang=_en

WHO. (2014). *Safe management of wastes from health-care activities*. World Health Organization.

WHO. (2018, February 8). *Health care waste fact sheet*. World Health Organization. Retrieved October 14, 2021, from https://www.who.int/news-room/fact-sheets/detail/heath-care-waste

WHO. (2021a). *Health-care waste key facts*. World Health Organisation. https://www.who.int/news-room/fact-sheets/detail/health-care-waste

WHO. (2021b). *WHO, Coronavirus (COVID-19) dashboard*. World Health Organization. Retrieved October 15, 2021, from https://covid19.who.int/

Zafar, S. (2019). Medical waste managment in developing countries. In T. S.-K. Winter Franz & S. T.-K. Thiel (Eds.), *Waste management, volume 9, waste to energy* (Vol. 9). Thomé-Kozmiensky Verlag GmbH.

9 Pandemic-Associated Biomedical Waste Management

Socio-Environmental Impact, Sustainable Strategies, and Renewable Technologies

Chockaiyan Usha, Parameswaran Kiruthika Lakshmi, Pandi Sakthieaswari, Mani Lakshmi, and Nithiya Anbuselvam

9.1 INTRODUCTION

Globally, it is estimated that at least 4 million children die each year due to infectious diseases that are caused by unmanaged medical waste. Biomedical wastes (BMWs) are the prospective cause of the foremost hazardous environmental pollutants. If not properly handled, BMW may carry a high amount of pathogenicity

DOI: 10.1201/9781003499695-9

and can cause severe health problems (Ilyas et al., 2020). The World Health Organization (2017) reported that BMW includes all the waste from medical procedures in healthcare facilities, research centres, and diagnostic laboratories. BMW also includes waste produced during any healthcare activities that take place at home. The types and characteristics of the contents determine the hazardous nature of the BMW. The classification of BMW is based on the existence of infectious substances; the presence of sharps; genotoxic, cytotoxic, and other toxic chemicals; and biologically violent pharmaceuticals. In India, to deal with the troubles associated with BMW, under the Environment (Protection) Act 1986 provision, Bio-Medical Waste (Management and Handling) Rules, 1998 was notified. These regulations pertain to all persons who accumulate, collect, accumulate, transfer, take care of, and dispose of BMW. Later, it was revised (2016) and subsequently amended (2018) to further advance the segregation, transportation, and disposal of BMW with reduced environmental impact (BMWM Rules, 2018). The COVID-19 pandemic has produced a global health tragedy along with varied impacts on the environment, economy, and general public. It has challenged the existing policy and BMW management practices (Choudhury et al., 2022). Wuhan City in China witnessed an increase in BMW generation by 600% in the middle of the COVID-19 outbreak (Jiajun, 2020). Constraints in recycling to prevent the increase of viruses and improper treatment have posed distressing conditions (Misra et al., 2020). The management of BMW during the COVID situation has been considered a foremost concern by numerous researchers (Boora et al., 2020; Misra et al., 2020), which can boost the threat of additional infection. As the increased generation of BMW is anticipated during the COVID-19 outbreak, secure usage, treatment, and waste discarding must be considered to minimize land, water, and air contamination. Studies from Tehran report that there is an undeniable link between the number of COVID-infected patients and the BMW generated (Ramteke & Sahu, 2020). India was reported to be the second-highest country with respect to people affected by the coronavirus. Kaur (2020) reported that India has crossed the saturation stage of available discarding facilities. The figure in the United States has grown considerably from 5 million tons annually to 2.5 million tons monthly (Ilyas et al., 2020). Considering the earlier incidences of pandemics, it has been found that SARS-CoV-2 spreads more quickly than the prior outbreaks from the same coronavirus family. Healthcare workers were the major infected populations at elevated rates due to the pandemic conditions. When Zika virus cases were found in Brazil in 2015, the World Health Organization gave instant regulations to restrain the virus by spreading information. Also, it strengthened healthcare facilities (WHO, 2017). Improper BMW management results in several problems, including the spread of the disease and environmental pollution (Rai et al., 2020). It has been recognized that 10–25% of BMW is hazardous and also reported to pose physical, chemical, and/or microbiological threats to persons exposed or associated in handling and treating waste (Rao & Ghosh, 2020). The report of the Special

Rapporteur UN Human Rights Council examines the undesirable effects that the improper management and disposal of BMW may have on the public and recommends additional measures that relevant stakeholders can consider to make improvements in the environmentally safe management and disposal of BMW (Human Rights Council-United Nations, 2011). However, there is a vital need for the reconstruction of management frameworks considering socio–economic–environmental feasibility. This chapter begins with a discussion of the existing problems and policy gaps associated with BMW, followed by environmental and social impact, concerns and conditions of operation in suburbs and remote areas, strategies for waste management, and the role of municipalities and NGOs. The chapter concludes by discussing renewable energy and nano-based technologies.

9.2 SOURCES AND TYPES OF BIOMEDICAL WASTE

The main sources of BMW are derived from hospitals, medical clinics, laboratories, and pharmaceutical factories. Other sources include blood donation camps, slaughterhouses, cosmetic services, vaccination centres, and funeral services (Table 9.1). BMWs can be categorized based on their origin and physical, chemical, or biological characteristics. Figure 9.1 and Table 9.1 illustrate the types and categorization of biomedical wastes.

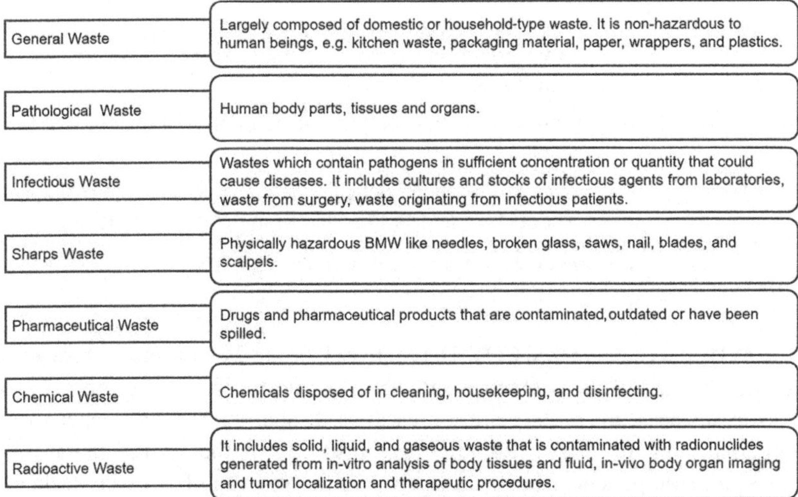

FIGURE 9.1 Types and categorization of biomedical wastes.

TABLE 9.1 Sources and Categorization of Biomedical Wastes

CATEGORY	*SOURCES OF BIOMEDICAL WASTES*
1	Human anatomical waste (human tissues, organs, body parts)
2	Animal waste (animal tissues, organs, body parts, carcasses, bleeding parts, fluid, blood, experimental animals used in research, waste generated by veterinary hospitals, colleges, discharge from hospitals, animal houses)
3	Microbiology and biotechnology waste (laboratory cultures, stocks or specimens of micro-organisms, live or attenuated vaccines, human and animal cell cultures used in research and industrial laboratories, wastes from production of biological products, dishes and devices used for transfer of cultures)
4	Waste sharps (needles, syringes, scalpels, blades, glass, that may cause puncture and unused sharps)
5	Discarded medicines and cytotoxic drugs (wastes comprising outdated, contaminated, and discarded medicines)
6	Soiled waste (items contaminated with blood and body fluids, including cotton, dressings, soiled plaster casts, lines, beddings, other material contaminated with blood)
7	Solid waste (wastes generated from disposable items other than waste sharps such as tabbing, catheters, intravenous sets)
8	Liquid waste (waste generated from laboratories and washing, cleaning, housekeeping, and disinfecting activities)
9	Incineration ash (ash from incineration of any bio-medical waste)
10	Chemical waste (chemicals used in production of biological products, chemicals used in disinfection, insecticides)

(*Source:* Biomedical wastes (Management and Handling Rules, 1998)).

WHO has categorized COVID-19 into risk group 2 on the bio-hazard level as the COVID-19 virus remains infectious for up to 72 hours on metal and plastic surfaces, up to 24 hours on cardboard, and 4 hours on copper (Van Doremalen et al., 2020). Research has also shown that symptomatic and asymptomatic patients can shed the virus in faeces even after being declared cured (ISWA-Netherlands, 2020).

9.3 EXISTING PROBLEMS WITH BMW

A major issue related to current BMW management in many hospitals is that the implementation of biomedical waste regulation is unsatisfactory, as some hospitals are disposing of waste in a haphazard, improper, and indiscriminate manner. Lack of segregation practices results in mixing of hospital wastes with general waste, making the whole waste stream hazardous. Inappropriate segregation ultimately results in an incorrect method of waste disposal. Inadequate biomedical waste management thus will cause environmental pollution; unpleasant smells; and growth and multiplication of vectors like insects, rodents, and worms and may lead to the transmission of diseases like typhoid, cholera, hepatitis, and AIDS through injuries from syringes and needles contaminated with human waste. The need for a proper hospital waste management system is of prime importance and is an essential component of quality assurance in hospitals. Figure 9.2 provides a summarized presentation of BMW-associated safety measures to be followed at quarantine centres.

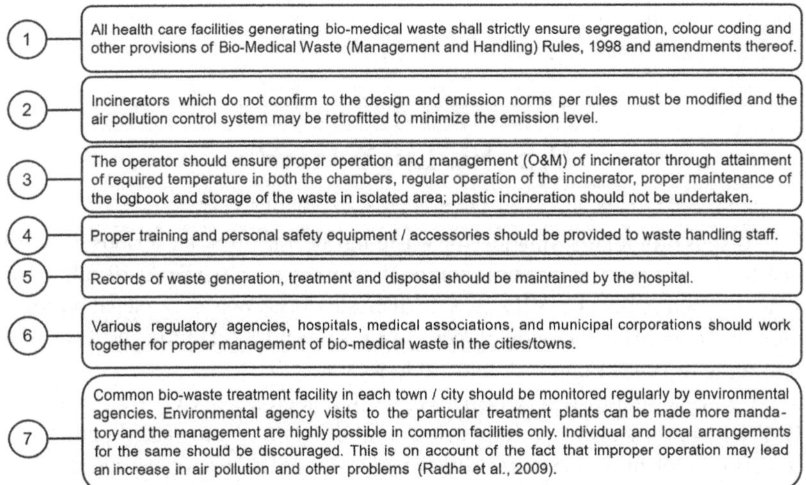

FIGURE 9.2 Measures to follow at quarantine centres.

9.4 MANAGING LIQUID WASTE AND WASTEWATER FROM HOSPITALS AND LABORATORIES

Wastewater refers to any water whose quality has been compromised by human activities. It includes liquid waste discharged from domestic homes, agricultural commercial sectors, pharmaceutical sectors, and hospitals. Hospital wastewater can contain hazardous substances, such as pharmaceutical residues, chemical hazardous substances, pathogens, and radioisotopes. Due to these substances, hospital wastewater can represent a chemical, biological, and physical risk for public and environmental health. Nevertheless, very frequently there are no legal requirements for hospital effluent treatment prior to its discharge into the municipal collector or directly onto surface water after pretreatment. Antibiotic-resistant organisms enter water environments from human and animal sources. These bacteria are able to spread their genes into water-indigenous microbes, which also contain resistance genes. On the contrary, many antibiotics from industrial origin circulate in water environments, potentially altering microbial ecosystems. Methods to reduce resistant bacterial load in wastewaters, and the amount of antimicrobial agents, in most cases originating from hospitals and farms, include optimization of disinfection procedures and management of wastewater and manure. A policy for preventing mixing human-originated and animal-originated bacteria with environmental organisms seems advisable.

9.5 POLICY GAPS

Safe disposal of a large quantity of waste has become a more serious concern due to the widespread transmission of the coronavirus (COVID-19) globally. After the outbreak of COVID-19, safe disposal of BMW is now a legal requirement in India. The Biomedical Waste Management & Handling Rules came into force in 1998 (Figure 9.3 and Table 9.4).

Central Pollution Control Board (CPCB) guidelines on COVID-19–related BMW management instructed various authorities to train waste handlers on infection prevention measures, hand hygiene, and respiratory etiquette. The CPCB also created audio-visual awareness material for related stakeholders (CPCB, 2020). Waste disposal staff and frontline workers should be adequately trained and protective equipment regularly provided. Globally, most workers employed in waste disposal and treatment plants are poor, so the common people also should come forward to provide protective kits free of cost, which may protect them from infection.

Schedule I	Categories of Biomedical Wastes.
Schedule II	Color Coding and Type of Container for Disposal of Biomedical Wastes.
Schedule III	Label for Biomedical Waste Containers / Bags.
Schedule IV	Label for Transportation of Biomedical Wastes.
Schedule V	Standards for Disposal and Treatment of Biomedical Waste Standards for Incinerators.
Schedule VI	Schedule for Waste Treatment Facilities like Incinerators/Autoclave/Microwave Systems.

FIGURE 9.3 Six schedules of biomedical waste management.

Source: The Biomedical Waste (Management and Handling) Rules, 199

Color Coding	Type of Container	Waste Category	Types of Disposal
Yellow	Plastic Bag Disinfected	1, 2, 3, 6	Incineration / Deep Burial
Red	Disinfected Container / Plastic Bags	3, 6, 7	Autoclaving / Microwaving / Chemical Treatment
Blue / White Translucent	Plastic Bags / Puncture Proof Container	4, 7	Autoclaving / Microwaving / Chemical Treatment Destruction / Shredding
Black	Plastic Bag	5, 9, 10 (Solids)	Disposal in Second Landfill

TABLE 9.4 Schedule II—Colour Coding and Type of Container for BMW Disposal

9.6 ENVIRONMENTAL AND SOCIAL IMPACT

A healthy environment is the most important factor in having a healthy lifestyle. Healthcare waste is the second most hazardous waste in the world, after radiation waste. The trash generated in many hospitals is linked to the human environment, either directly or indirectly (WHO, 2018). Non-hazardous waste, pathological waste, radioactive waste, infectious waste, chemical waste, cytotoxic waste, sharps waste, and pharmaceutical waste are all examples of medical trash and its derivatives (Rodriguez-Morales, 2013).

9.6.1 Open Dumping

A landfill is a structure designed to bury solid waste in the earth, and open dumps are the most basic type of landfill. COVID-19 has resulted in a significant increase in the creation of BMW. India produced roughly 600 tonnes of BMW every day before the outbreak. The country created 203 tonnes of COVID-related garbage per day in May when the second wave was at its peak. The negative consequences of unlawful medical waste dumping are eye-opening, alarming, and disappointing. Human dangers are simply drawbacks of incorrect medical waste disposal techniques. Severe environmental destruction is also a problem. The potential of hazardous particles, poisons, or other contaminants entering the environment increases when BMW is not properly treated. Even the most advanced water treatment plants and sewage collecting systems cannot eliminate all contaminants from wastewater, such as bacteria or medications, leaving traces of substances that could be released into the environment. Despite the Health Department's explicit instructions, the danger of discarding biomedical waste in the open persists.

9.6.2 Marine Litter

The problem of marine trash is global in scope and has an intergenerational impact. Any humanmade, manufactured, or processed waste discarded, disposed of, or abandoned in the maritime environment is referred to as marine debris or marine litter. COVID-induced behavioural change is worsening the problem of ocean pollution as the world battles to deal with the ongoing COVID-19 epidemic. Some countries have attempted to make reusable masks more widely available; nonetheless, most people still rely on single-use medical masks and latex gloves. These abandoned masks and gloves, along with other human trash, wind up in the ocean in alarming numbers of cases. Multiple surveys from nations worldwide have documented an increase in discarded single-use latex gloves and surgical masks washing up on beaches and coasts around the world.

9.6.3 Open Burning: Incineration Is a Public Health Concern

Pathogens can pollute the air we breathe outside. Pathogens can enter the atmosphere if BMW is transferred outside the institution without being pre-treated or deposited in open locations. There are two major sources of chemical pollutants that produce outdoor air pollution, open burning and incinerators. The most hazardous technique is the open burning of BMW. When inhaled, it can lead to respiratory problems. Dioxins and furans, for example, are carcinogenic organic gases. The design parameters and upkeep of treatment and disposal technology should adhere to the established guidelines. Incinerator and open-fire emissions expose people to hazardous gases that might cause cancer and respiratory ailments. The world's BMW management system has been put to the test due to COVID-19–induced pandemics.

9.6.4 Liquid Waste and Wastewater from Hospitals and Laboratories

The release of large amounts of antimicrobials in hospital wastewater initiates a continuous selective pressure that contributes to the proliferation of resistant microbes (Kraemer et al., 2019). Mismanagement of hospital waste, including wastewater, leads to the emergence and spread of antimicrobial-resistant bacteria. Clinical laboratories generate huge amounts of liquid infectious waste in the form of bodily fluids, such as blood. BMW is the term used to describe the solid waste created in healthcare facilities. In a hospital, liquid-infected waste management is mostly addressed in the form of a sewage treatment plant or an effluent treatment plant, both of which are required. The construction of these facilities necessitates a significant financial investment. Smaller facilities may be unable to afford to build an STP on their premises.

9.6.5 Concern with Conditions of Operation in Suburbs and Remote Areas

COVID-19 has caused a global health crisis with many economic, societal, and environmental consequences. Efforts to battle the pandemic have resulted in a major increase in BMW production. Telehealth can help healthcare systems, organizations, and clinicians increase access to and quality of care in rural areas. Using telehealth to deliver and assist with delivering healthcare services in remote locations can help patients overcome hurdles and burdens, such as transportation issues, while traveling for specialty care. Telehealth can also improve monitoring, timeliness, and communications within the healthcare system. Telehealth initiatives can be used as models for developing and implementing telehealth programs in rural hospitals and clinics. Workforce issues, quality of care concerns, reimbursement, licensure, and availability to internet services are all challenges that can be prepared for when offering telehealth services in rural locations (WHO, 2020).

9.6.6 Landfill Sites: A Source of Leachate of Water

Landfills have been identified as one of the biggest hazards to groundwater resources in India and worldwide (United States Environmental Protection Agency). Over 90% of India's municipal solid waste (MSW) is inadequately dumped on land. The waste dumped in landfills or open dumps is exposed to groundwater underflow, precipitation infiltration, and other water infiltration. Leachate is a liquid that contains a variety of organic and inorganic chemicals (Mondal et al., 2023). This leachate collects at the landfill's bottom, percolates through the earth, and eventually reaches the groundwater. Because of the potential polluting source of leachate originating from the local dumping site, areas around landfills have a higher risk of groundwater contamination. Groundwater contamination poses a significant concern to local groundwater resource users and the natural environment. There are a variety of ways to assess the contamination of groundwater and surface water.

It can be determined by experimentally measuring contaminants or estimating them using mathematical modelling (EPA, 2021). All people who support and finance healthcare activities have a social and legal duty for the safe and sustainable management of BMW. The approach is to build additional BMW treatment facilities in areas where they are sorely needed and to use a carrot-and-stick policy to ensure that hospitals obey waste disposal requirements. Furthermore, much research and development are required in the field of producing environmentally friendly medical devices and BMW disposal systems to achieve a greener and cleaner environment (Datta, 2018).

9.7 DEVELOPING RESILIENCE AND PREPAREDNESS FOR EVENTS IN THE FUTURE BY REDESIGNING WASTE MANAGEMENT SYSTEMS

The COVID-19 pandemic has already had a huge impact on the garbage industry. Initially, as the pandemic spread and several countries implemented lockdowns, public authorities and municipal trash operators had to quickly adjust their waste management systems and procedures to the circumstances. The scientific community has been working to examine the virus, its socio-environmental effects, regulatory or adaptation policies, and plans from the beginning of the COVID-19 issue. The emergency is to build pandemic-resilient municipal design and administration to combat infectious diseases. Such development entails re-framing unsustainable urban patterns, risks, and socio-economic disparities to prepare for upcoming scenarios (Sarkodie, 2020).

9.7.1 Capacity Building of Sanitation Workers

Sanitation employees help communities by collecting rubbish and transporting it to appropriate disposal sites such as dumps or landfills. The worldwide sanitation workforce is responsible for bridging the gap between sanitation infrastructure and sanitation services. Sanitation workers provide an important public service, but they often sacrifice their dignity, safety, health, and living conditions in the process. They are among the most precarious workers. Public awareness raises public knowledge of issues and mobilizes popular support and action. Public events, workshops, exhibitions, demonstrations, radio and television campaigns, print publications, and the Internet are all examples of how it might be done (Dalberg, 2017).

9.7.2 Role of Municipalities and NGOs

A second phase begins as the lockdown or other restrictive restrictions gradually ease, and new obstacles emerge. Public authorities and municipal trash operators do not need to act in an emergency. Still, they must now deal with the consequences of the various steps taken in the so-called first phase and the need to analyse the situation. As national governments and development partners strive toward attaining properly managed sanitation for all, all stakeholders have a role in protecting sanitation workers' dignity, health, and lives. Development partners, NGOs, and civil society can increase awareness of sanitation workers' public service and misery and campaign for their health, safety, dignity, and rights at the global, national, and subnational levels. Supporting worker unions, professional organizations, development partners, NGOs, and civil society may help sanitation employees assert their rights.

9.7.3 Renewable Energy Technologies

Waste management, which involves the responsible collection, transportation, processing, and disposal of hazardous and non-hazardous waste material, is an important aspect of the environmental protection. The efficient management of biological waste is a particular concern. Waste to Energy (WtE) technology is an energy recovery process that turns leftover waste chemicals into useful forms of energy such as electricity, heat, or steam. Thermal conversion techniques are now the most used WtE technology. The systemic approach for BMW regarding a chain of environmental and health risks and concerns can be followed (EPA, 2021).

9.7.4 Nano-Based Technologies

The COVID-19 outbreak has spurred a global desire for efficient diagnosis and treatment and infection mitigation through large-scale measures like alternate antiviral treatments and traditional disinfection protocols. Using nanotechnology opens new possibilities for developing revolutionary COVID-19 and other viral infection prevention, diagnosis, and treatment procedures.

Nanotechnology-based methods could be used in pandemic diagnosis, prevention, and treatment. They offer several techniques to deal with this situation, based on an abundance of designed materials identified by their relevant physicochemical features through diverse chemical functionalization. COVID-19 and infectious diseases in general, including future pandemics, can benefit from nanotechnology-based therapies. Nanotechnology has the potential to facilitate the development of simple, rapid, and cost-effective nanotechnology-based assays to monitor the presence of SARS-CoV-2 and related biomarkers, in addition to disease prevention and therapeutic potential. Nanostructured drug development and delivery-based research and development are now promising the globe to drastically improve therapeutic, diagnostic, and prevention options to stop epidemics effectively and quickly. If all regulatory, scale-up, and safety challenges are resolved, nanotechnology has the potential to protect the globe from the current and future pandemic crises.

REFERENCES

Bio-medical waste management (Amendment) rules. (2018). https://pcb.ap.gov.in/APPCBDOCS/Tenders_Noti/WasteManagement/Bio%20medical%20waste%20management%20(amendment)%20Rules%202018.pdf

Boora, S., Gulia, S. K., Kausar, M., Tadia, V. K., Choudhary, A. H., & Lathwal, A. (2020). Role of hospital administration department in managing Covid-19 pandemic in India. *Journal of Advanced Medical and Dental Sciences Research, 8*(5).

Choudhury, M., Sahoo, S., Samanta, P., Tiwari, A., Tiwari, A., Tiwari, A., Chadha, U., & Chakravorty, A. (2022). COVID-19: An accelerator for global plastic consumption and its implications. *Journal of Environmental and Public Health, 2022*. https://doi.org/10.1155/2022/1066350

CPCB. (2020). *Guidelines for handling, treatment, and disposal of waste generated during treatment/diagnosis/quarantine of COVID-19 Patients—Rev. 4*. Central Pollution Control Board. Government of India.

Dalberg Advisor. (2017). *Sanitation worker safety and livelihoods in India: A blueprint for action*. https://www.susana.org/_resources/documents/default/3-3483-7-15427-26162.pdf

Datta, P., Mohi, G. K., & Chander, J. (2018). Biomedical waste management in India: Critical appraisal. *Journal of Laboratory Physicians, 10*, 6–14.

Environmental and health risks and concerns. (2021). Environmental Protection Agency. https://www.epa.gov/climateimpacts/climate-change-and-human-health

Gursimran Kaur Mohi, Bhavana Yadav, Ishani Bora et.al. Biomedical waste management during COVID-19 pandemic: a medical institute perspective. *Int J Health Sci Res*. 2023; *13*(2), 98–104. DOI: https://doi.org/10.52403/ijhsr.20230216

Human Rights Council, United Nations. (2011, July 4). Report of the special rapporteur on the adverse effects of the movement and dumping of toxic and dangerous products and wastes on the enjoyment of human rights. *Calin Georgescu*, 18th Session. https://www.ohchr.org/en/statements/2011/10/statement-mr-calin-georgescu-special-rapporteur-toxics-and-human-rights

Ilyas, S., Srivastava, R. R., & Kim, H. (2020). Disinfection technology and strategies for COVID-19 hospital and bio-medical waste management. *Science of the Total Environment*, 141652.

ISWA-Netherlands. (2020). *Country specific waste management responses, COVID-19 response international knowledge sharing on waste management*. https://www.iswa.org/fileadmin/galleries/0001_COVID/Jordan_Solid_Waste_Handling_Manual_Coronavirus_crisis-ENG.pdf

Jiajun, W. (2020). *Cement industry in China assisted with disposal of Covid-19 healthcare waste*. https://www.zkg.de/en/artikel/zkg_Cement_industry_in_China_assisted_with_disposal_of_Covid-19_healthcare_%203535100.html

Kraemer, S. A., Ramachandran, A., & Perron, G. G. (2019). Antibiotic pollution in the environment: From microbial ecology to public policy. *Microorganisms*, *7*(6), 180.

Misra, V., Bhardwaj, A., Bhardwaj, S., & Misra, S. (2020). Novel COVID-19–Origin, emerging challenges, recent trends, transmission routes and Control-A review. *Journal of Contemporary Orthodontics*, *4*(1), 55–56.

Mondal, T., Choudhury, M., Kundu, D., Dutta, D., & Samanta, P. (2023). Landfill: An eclectic review on structure, reactions and remediation approach. *Waste Management*, *164*, 127–142. https://doi.org/10.1016/j.wasman.2023.03.034

Rai, A., Kothari, R., & Singh, D. P. (2020). Assessment of available technologies for hospital waste management: A need for society. In *Waste management:* Concepts, *methodologies, tools, and applications* (pp. 860–876). IGI Global.

Ramteke, S., & Sahu, B. L. (2020). Novel coronavirus disease 2019 (COVID-19) pandemic: Considerations for the biomedical waste sector in India. *CSCEE*, *1*, 100029.

Rao, V. V., & Ghosh, S. K. (2020). Sustainable bio medical waste management—case study in India. In *Urban mining and sustainable Waste management* (pp. 303–317). Springer.

Sarkodie, S. A., & Owusu, P. A. (2020). Impact of COVID-19 pandemic on waste management. *Environment, Development and Sustainability*, 1–10.

Van Doremalen, N., Bushmaker, T., Morris, D. H., Holbrook, M. G., Gamble, A., Williamson, B. N., Tamin, A., Harcourt, J. L., Thornburg, N. J., Gerber, S. I., Lloyd-Smith, J. O., de Wit, E., & Munster, V. J. (2020). Aerosol and surface stability of SARS-CoV-2 as compared with SARS-CoV-1. *The New England Journal of Medicine*, *382*(16), 1564–1567.

WHO Health-care waste. (2018). https://www.who.int/news-room/fact-sheets/detail/health-care-waste

World Health Organization. (2017). *Report on health-care waste management (HCWM) status in countries of the South-East Asia region (No. SEA-EH-593)*. World Health Organization. Regional Office for South-East Asia.

World Health Organization. (2020). *Water, sanitation, hygiene, and waste management for SARS-COV-2, the virus that causes Covid-19*. https://www.who.int/publications/i/item/WHO-2019-nCoV-IPC-WASH-2020.4

10 Environmental Concerns and Recent Advances in Management of Pandemic-Associated Biomedical Wastes

Case Studies on India and Bangladesh

Palas Samanta, Sukhendu Dey, Apurba Ratan Ghosh, and Md. Moniruzzaman

10.1 INTRODUCTION

COVID-19 has affected the whole world since its emergence in December 2019 and has been declared a Public Health Emergency of International Concern (PHEIC) (Samanta et al., 2021). During the COVID-19 lockdown period, humanity

DOI: 10.1201/9781003499695-10

experienced a clean environment with reduced air pollution levels, relatively healthy water, decreased environmental noise, improved soil fertility, and striking growth in biodiversity. However, there were several negative aspects like increased hospitalizations; complete isolation at home; and an increase in the use of personal protective equipment, disposable life support systems, healthcare devices, and other medical protective gear that are made up of non-biodegradable substances (Rahman et al., 2020). Stockpiling of this personal protective equipment and medical items caused a health emergency due to unwanted and uncontrolled waste generation from healthcare facilities and households (De-la-Torre et al., 2021). Environmental degradation due to accelerated waste production and inappropriate disposal was a global challenge even before COVID-19 (Boucher & Billard, 2019). COVID-19 has altered both qualitative and quantitative aspects of waste management, thus leading to environmental degradation (Shammi & Tareq, 2021). Mismanagement of contaminated wastes from domestic and healthcare facilities accelerated the spread of COVID-19 infection through secondary transmission. Thus, the sustainable management of healthcare-associated wastes is a big challenge (Boucher & Billard, 2019). The developing countries lacking standard protocols and guidelines for pandemic-associated biomedical waste management are more likely to face adverse public health consequences. The chapter deals with the concerns, challenges, and recent advancements associated with COVID-19–associated biomedical waste management. The chapter begins by discussing the impact of COVID-19–associated BMW on the surrounding environment, animal and human health, and their interconnectedness. It concisely points out the perspectives of the Central Pollution Control Board (India), the World Health Organization (WHO), OSHA (USA), the European Union (EU), and the National System for Environmental Protection (NSEP). This will be followed by coverage of bioremediation strategies for COVID-19–associated BMW and conclude with an analysis of the scenario in India and Bangladesh. The chapter focuses on addressing SDG 3 (Good Health and Wellbeing), SDG 6 (Clean Water and Sanitation), SDG 7 (Clean and Affordable Energy), SDG 8 (Decent Work and Economic Growth), SDG 9 (Industry, Innovation, and Infrastructure), SDG 10 (Reduced Inequalities), SDG 11 (Sustainable Cities and Communities), SDG 12 (Responsible Consumption and Production), SDG 14 (Life Below Water), SDG 15 (Life on Land), SDG 16 (Peace, Justice, and Strong Institutions), and SDG 17 (Partnerships for the Goals).

10.2 ENVIRONMENTAL CONCERNS OF COVID-19 WASTE

The mismanagement of pandemic-associated waste adversely affects every sector of the environment, including human beings. Additionally, the non-biodegradable nature of COVID-19 waste has accelerated the consequences. The effects of poor handling and mismanagement of waste are categorized into three classes: the impact on animals, humans, and the environment.

10.2.1 Effects on Animal Health

Improper waste management adversely affects various animals, including fish, birds, invertebrates, mammals, turtles, and reptiles, by entanglement or ingestion. Plastic-associated wastes affect the respiratory system, developmental activities, foraging, movement, and reproduction (Kögel et al., 2020). Under long-term effects, COVID-19–related wastes adversely affect the food chain/food web of aquatic ecosystems and finally threaten humans (Choi et al., 2020). Additionally, COVID-19 wastes can trap/carry different kinds of toxic/hazardous substances ranging from additives to plasticizers, which ultimately pose a threat to public health and the environment. Upon bioaccumulation, these contaminants cross the cell membrane and finally create different physiological burdens and immunological disorders in humans due to their retention in blood, the brain, and the placenta (Goodman et al., 2021). Researchers documented that inhalation or ingestion of PPE-derived micro/meso/nano-plastics results in teratogenic responses, cellular membrane permeability, and pulmonary disorders through in vitro and in vivo observations on wild animals (Shi et al., 2021).

PPE-derived micro/meso/nano-plastics directly affect wildlife via entanglement or ingestion (Hiemstra et al., 2021). For example, Magellanic penguin death (*Spheniscus magellanicus*) from Brazil due to FFP-2 protective face mask ingestion has been reported by Neto et al. (2021). Boyle (2020) observed the death of a bird due to entanglement in a discarded coronavirus facemask in a tree. Lavers et al. (2020) reported entrapment of *Coenobita perlatus* in PPE-associated plastic litter. Several other authors documented death of wild animals such as peregrine falcons (*Falco peregrinus*), American robins (*Turdus migratorius*), seagulls (*Larus* sp.), swans (*Cygnus olor*), hedgehogs (*Erinaceus europaeus*), mallards (*Anas platyrhynchos*), bats (*Eptesicus serotinus*), foxes (*Vulpes vulpes*), crabs (*Carcinus maenas*), and checkered puffer fish (*Sphoeroides testudineus*) due to entanglement (legs, beak, talons, neck, or other body parts) in disposable COVID-19 face masks or litter (Hiemstra et al., 2021).

10.2.2 Effects on Human Health

COVID-19 pandemic–associated wastes have great potential to cause detrimental effects on the human body upon entry (Samanta & Ghosh, 2021).

COVID-19 wastes can spread the disease directly if poorly managed and disposed of. Prata et al. (2020) documented PPE-derived micro/meso/nano-plastic–induced lung inflammation in the human body. Prata et al. (2020) categorized PPE-derived micro/meso/nano-plastic health effects into three broad classes, inflammatory disorders, immune disorders, and neurodegeneration. The inhalation of PPE-derived micro/meso/nano-plastics caused severe health effects like chronic inflammation, DNA damage, cellular damage, oxidative stress, granulomas or fibrosis, and cytokine secretion (De-la-Torre et al., 2021). These adverse public health effects are accelerated severalfold due to the entry of hazardous substances like heavy metals, toxic microorganisms, pesticides, polycyclic aromatic hydrocarbons, additives, and plasticizers, as these wastes act as vector or carriers of contaminants (Torres et al., 2021). This contamination caused both primary as well as secondary adverse health outcomes such as physiological and reproductive disorders, digestive problems, respiratory disorders, impaired immunity, malignant cancers, endocrine disruption, leukaemia, birth difficulty, ophthalmologic responses, and even spreading of other communicable diseases (De-la-Torre et al., 2021).

10.2.3 Effects on Environmental Sectors

Several environmental issues can originate due to the generation of COVID-19 wastes and subsequent mismanagement, such as land, air, and water deterioration (Samanta & Ghosh, 2021). Online procurement systems due to stay-home practices have also accelerated household organic and inorganic waste generation. The poor handling and disposal of these wastes in the natural environment greatly altered the chemical composition of the land, particularly acidity and alkalinity. The dumping of PPE items irregularly causes toxicity to land due to their chemical degradation/decomposition (De-la-Torre et al., 2021). Upon degradation/decomposition, these PPE items generate huge amounts of macro/meso/micro/nano-plastics and become an environmental concern due to their easy penetration/transmission into environmental segments. They reduce the fertility of soil as well as productivity and ultimately cause different potential health problems. Finally, this land degradation caused a loss of biodiversity. Additionally, the soil containing active SARS-COV-2 virus can accelerate the spread of the disease as secondary transmission. PPE items contribute carbon dioxide (CO_2) into the environment, ultimately leading to global warming and climate change. During PPE production, a significant amount of CO_2 is released into the atmosphere. For example, a single face mask and surgical face mask released approximately 50 and 59 g CO_2-equivalent greenhouse gas emission (GHGs), respectively, into the environment, while a single cloth mask released about 60 g CO_2-equivalent GHG emission (Klemeš et al., 2020). According to an estimate, the United Kingdom alone could generate approx. 124,000 tons of plastic waste (unrecyclable) and 66,000 tons of contaminated waste if every individual disposes of one surgical mask per day over a year period (Allison et al., 2020). Kumar et al. (2020) documented that transportation of 10 tons of PPE items (about 10 km distance) to a disposal site released approximately 2.76 kg CO_2-equivalent global warming potential (GWP). Further, the incidence of acid rain and nosocomial infections could be common environmental consequences. Moreover, it can aid in the easy transfer and prevalence of other airborne diseases like pneumonia and tuberculosis (De-la-Torre et al., 2021). The water segment also received huge attention during the COVID-19 pandemic as dumping and incineration of PPE items caused an unprecedented impact on water quality or water resources. The improper disposal of PPE items containing the SARS-COV-2 virus has the potential to contaminate sewage water and waste water. In addition to this, water is polluted adversely due to the entry of additional toxicants along with plastic wastes such as heavy metals, pesticides, additives, plasticizers, and polycyclic aromatic hydrocarbons (PAHs). These pollutants degrade the water quality and finally cause toxicity in aquatic ecosystems and ultimately to humans (Bilal et al., 2020). Wang et al. (2005) demonstrated that SARS-COV-2 virus in dechlorinated tap water can survive up to 2 days and therefore have the potential to spread the disease. Consequently, Muthuraman and Lakshminarayanan (2021) demonstrated that the occurrence of the COVID-19 outbreak in Hong Kong was primarily due to leakage in sewage line, which ultimately caused severe health problems due to its replication in the gastrointestinal tract (GIT).

10.3 STRATEGIES ADOPTED BY COUNTRIES ACROSS THE GLOBE TO MANAGE COVID-19

The COVID-19 outbreak has dramatically accelerated household and healthcare waste generation across the globe. Different government authorities around the world have implemented and/or adopted different technologies for effective management of COVID-19 wastes. Based on guidelines and environmental safety legislation formulated by different authorities, the COVID waste has attracted special emphasis across countries, especially waste collection sectors, followed by waste segregation. Tables 10.1 and 10.2 illustrate guidelines formulated by different government authorities during the COVID-19 outbreak to handle the emerging circumstances.

TABLE 10.1 COVID-19 Waste Management Guidelines Formulated by Different Agencies

AGENCY NAME	*COVID-19 WASTE MANAGEMENT GUIDELINES*
Central Pollution Control Board (CPCB), India	Colour-coded bags/containers use for proper waste segregation. Temporary collection and storing of COVID waste before transferring to CBMWTF. General and/or non-hazardous waste disposal per solid waste disposal guidelines.
World Health Organisation (WHO)	Hazardous waste segregation from healthcare units in specific-coloured tubs. Onsite disposal of infectious wastes through temperature (high) treatment or by incineration/autoclaving. Non-hazardous items (waiting areas of health care facilities; HCFs) should be sealed in black bags. Should adopt controlled waste burning in the absence of waste removal facilities.
Occupational Safety and Health Administration (OSHA), USA	Sanitation workers should use typical PPE items to handle COVID waste. COVID biomedical waste should be managed in a regulated manner because COVID-19 infection is not under Category A.
European Union (EU)	Mandatory use of individual waste bag for all infected items like face masks, tissues, and gloves and proper sealing. Regular collection of waste bags, and keep them with general waste bags. No need for special collection of waste.
National System for Environmental Protection (NSPA)	Municipal waste categorization in two classes: T1 and T2. T1 (household solid waste contaminated by COVID-19 patients) waste collection in double-layered bags and subsequent sterilization (no need for source isolation). T2 (waste from quarantine areas/non–COVID-19 patients) should be collected by properly equipped sanitary workers in double-layered bags.

TABLE 10.2 Sustainable COVID-19 Waste Disposal Procedures during and after COVID-19 Pandemic.

Sources of Waste/Procedure Followed during Disposal		
Household waste	COVID-19 quarantine centre	Hospital waste
Sources of Segregation		
Recyclable waste/residual waste	Residual waste	Biohazard waste

Packaging		
Regular packaging/paper bags can be used as packaging material. The life span of the virus is shorter (a few hours) compared to that on plastics (up to 7 days)	Double packing of wastes in disposable bags.	Anti-puncture packaging is recommended for biohazard waste.
Labelling		
N/A	Labelled as "COVID-19 Waste".	Labelled as "COVID-19 Waste".
Resting Time		
72 h	72 h	N/A
Disinfection		
The resting time will disinfect the waste.	• Use of disinfectants such as 80% ethanol, 75% 2-propanol. • Resting time is as long as possible to make sure disinfection occurs naturally.	• Autoclaving. • Resting time is as long as possible to make sure disinfection occurs naturally.
Disposal		
• Recyclables through recycling units. • Residual waste to sanitary landfills or incineration.	• Incineration.	• Incineration.
Remarks		
• Due to the current situation of the pandemic, recycling units are less operational, so it is recommended to discharge recyclables according to the capacity of recycling units. It will prevent the piling up of waste. • Instead of door-to-door waste collection, collection at a common location will help during limited staff availability.	All waste is treated as residual waste.	Proper disposal will minimize the transmission of pathogens.

10.4 COVID-19 WASTE MANAGEMENT SCENARIO IN INDIA AND BANGLADESH

For management of biomedical wastes, the Ministry of Environment and Forests, Government of India (GOI), enacted the Biomedical Waste (Management and Handling) Rules 1998 all over India on 28 July 1998. The standards gave the biomedical waste (BMW) definition for immunization camps, blood gift camps, or social insurance exercises undertaken outside the medicinal services office. As per the BMW (Management and Handling) Rules 2016 and its amendments, biomedical wastes generated from COVID-19 patients and staff workers during screening, treatment, management, and immunization should be handled as follows: on-site pre-treatment of certain type of wastes, segregation gained much importance for healthcare facilities (HCF) wastes, collection, processing, treatment and disposal must be conducted per Common Biomedical Waste Treatment & Disposal Facility (CBMWTF). The detailed guidelines that India is currently following are described in Table 10.3.

TABLE 10.3 Guidelines Followed by Indian Government to Handle COVID-19 Waste

WASTE CATEGORY	*COLOUR CODE*	*PRE-TREATMENT TYPE*	*DISPOSAL METHOD*
Blood, body fluid/ cotton swab–contaminated soiled waste	Yellow	Not required	Incineration
Laboratory chemicals, lab wastes, infected secretions, floor washing, aspirated body fluids, disinfection activities	Yellow	Separate collection, neutralization at ETPs	General draining
PPE items like face masks, face shields, gowns, caps, goggles	Yellow	Not necessary	Incineration
Discarded linen, blood/body fluid–contaminated bedding	Yellow	Not necessary	Disinfection (non-chlorinated) followed by incineration

WASTE CATEGORY	*COLOUR CODE*	*PRE-TREATMENT TYPE*	*DISPOSAL METHOD*
Lab and microbial waste like culture tubes, stocks, vaccines, specimens, devices	Yellow	Auto-clave, microwave, hydroclave, disinfection of plastic bag/ container by non-chlorine chemical	Pre-treatment and then incineration
Blood/body fluid–contaminated gloves	Red	Not necessary	Auto-clave/shredding and then recycling
IV tubing, catheters, bottles, vacutainers, urine bags	Red	Not necessary	Auto-clave/shredding and then recycling
Broken glassware, vials, ampules (no cytotoxic contamination)	Blue	Not required	Chemical disinfection followed by recycling
Scalpels, needles, blades, syringes (metallic sharp waste)	White	Not required	Auto-clave/shredding followed by encapsulation/ disposal in iron foundries

According to a Central Pollution Control Board report, during the COVID-19 pandemic, India is currently producing approximately 600 metric tons of BMW/day, which is about 10% higher than normal years (CPCB, 2020). It has also been estimated that each and every state of India is producing about 2 tons of COVID waste due to analyses, isolation, and COVID-19 treatment. The value is excessively low compared with 240 tons of COVID-19 waste/ day by the Wuhan province of China, the focal point of the pandemic (CPCB, 2020). To deal with COVID-19 waste, the Central Pollution Control Board, an autonomous institution of the government of India, released guidelines on 18 March 2020. According to these guidelines, isolation wards in HCFs should use discrete colour-coded canisters for controlled isolation of waste materials. Additionally, the buckets/dustbins should be marked "COVID-19" and must be placed in a separate space and given special care (CPCB, 2020). Further, separate strategies for sanitation workers/labourers in COVID-19 wards should be employed for biomedical waste administration. The guidelines also suggested keeping waste generation records in segregation wards. The guidelines further suggested that waste generated from isolation camps and home quarantine should be sorted into yellow packets, and canisters collecting these wastes should be handed over to the appropriate/concerned authorities. The standards also instructed that healthcare staff handling these wastes should have proper training and must wear PPE items like splash-proof aprons, masks (three-layered), gloves, goggles, and gumboots (CPCB, 2020). Apart from this, the CPCB also installed a COVID-19 BWM tracking app to monitor COVID-19–related BMW generation. Per data from June 2021, about 164 tons COVID-19–related biomedical waste are generated per day, there are about 13,000 COVID-19 waste generators, and about 198 CBMWTFs are working to manage high-volume COVID-19 waste.

Waste management including COVID-19 waste in countries like Bangladesh has become a challenging issue, particularly in urban areas, as 29.4% of the people (total 160 million people) in Bangladesh live in urban areas. Actually, uncontrolled dumpsites in Bangladesh create a burden on the environmental sector, including human health. Currently, Amin bazar and the Matuail area are used for dumping wastes for Dhaka city. The Bangladeshi government drafted a constitution regarding medical waste generation in 2008; despite this, no procurement management has been established to deal with healthcare waste created on a regular basis in hospitals, clinics, and homes. Wastes produced inside HCFs is frequently collected without sorting by inexperienced and unprotected sanitary workers and finally discarded in unapproved locations without appropriate treatment (Barua & Hossain, 2021). With the global spread of the SARS-CoV-2 virus, biomedical waste has emerged as challenging issue for human health, including the environment. Bangladesh already had poor waste management practices before the COVID-19 outbreak and has now been adversely affected by an unexpected surge in medical waste volume (Shammi & Tareq, 2021). To date, 654 government and 5055 private hospitals in Bangladesh are working very hard to tackle the COVID pandemic, altogether generating an enormous amount of biomedical waste. The average daily waste generation is about 1.63–1.99 kg per bed in Dhaka city. Accordingly, failure to handle this huge medical waste surge amid COVID-19 is likely to putt Bangladesh at further risk (Rahman et al., 2020). In addition to this, municipal solid waste management (MSWM) is another momentous issue in Bangladesh. Increased waste from municipal households and its arbitrary disposal led to environmental pollution. Further, during the pandemic, online shopping and delivery accelerated the generation of vast amounts of household waste. The use of gloves, masks, and other protective equipment at home to get rid from virus infection also increases the amount of harmful health waste generation. During the pandemic, the urban centres combined produced approximately 23,688 tons/day MSW, out of which 70% was organic solid waste (OSW) (Alam & Qiao, 2020). On the other hand, household solid wastes (HSW) constituted approximately 90% of the total MSW streams, out of which 80% – 92% was OSW (Alam & Qiao, 2020).

10.5 FUTURE RECOMMENDATIONS

Although several guidelines have been formulated across the globe to manage COVID-19 waste, the ongoing pandemic represents accelerated environmental consequences in waste generation from different sectors, especially HCFs and household units. Waste collection from these units should follow the prescribed government guidelines and subsequent treatment before disposal. The incineration technique is highly recommended for COVID outbreak peak areas, whereas deep burying of infectious waste is adopted for remote areas facing in situ facilities. Untrained/unskilled personnel/sanitation staff should not be engaged in COVID-19 waste handling specifically during segregation of wastes, as they are very contagious and have the potential to infect them with different pathogens like tuberculosis or HIV. Therefore, mass awareness of healthcare staff is mandatory for effective management of this kind of contagious waste. Additionally, government authorities should adopt technologies to handle COVID-19 waste such as waste-to-energy recovery technologies like recycling and bioremediation.

REFERENCES

Alam, O., & Qiao, X. (2020). An in-depth review on municipal solid waste management, treatment and disposal in Bangladesh. *Sustain Cities Society*, *52*, 101775. https://doi.org/10.1016/j.scs.2019.101775

Allison, A.L., Ambrose-Dempster, E., Domenech Aparsi, T., Bawn, M., Casas Arredondo, M., Chau, C., Chandler, K., Dobrijevic, D., Hailes, H., Lettieri, P., Liu, C., Medda, F., Michie, S., Miodownik, M., Purkiss, D., & Ward, J. (2020). *The environmental dangers of employing single-use face masks as part of a COVID-19 exit strategy* (UCL Open: Environment Preprint). UCL Press.

Barua, U., & Hossain, D. (2021). A review of the medical waste management system at Covid-19 situation in Bangladesh. *Journal of Material Cycles and Waste Management*, 1–14.

Bilal, M, Mehmood, S., & Iqbal, H. (2020). The beast of beauty: Environmental and health concerns of toxic components in cosmetics. *Cosmetics*, *7*(1), 13.

Boucher, J., & Billard, G. (2019). The challenges of measuring plastic pollution. Field Actions Science Reports, SI19:68–75. IUCN. *Review of Plastic Footprint*

Methodologies. portals.iucn.org/library/sites/library/files/documents/2019-027-En.pdf

Boyle, L. (2020). Bird dies after getting tangled in coronavirus face mask. *Independent New York*. https://www.independent.co.uk/climate-change/news/coronavirus-face-mask-bird-death-recycle-environment-conservation-a9475341.html

Central Pollution Control Board CPCB. (2020). *Guidelines for handling, treatment and disposal of waste generated during treatment/diagnosis/quarantine of COVID-19 patients*. Central Pollution Control Board, Govt. of India.

Choi, D., Bang, J., Kim, T., Oh, Y., Hwang, Y., & Hong, J. (2020). In vitro chemical and physical toxicities of polystyrene micro-fragments in human-derived cells. *Journal of Hazardous Materials*, *400*, 123308

De-la-Torre, G. E., Pizarro-Ortega, C. I., Dioses-Salinas, D. C., Ammendolia, J., & Okoffo, E. D. (2021). Investigating the current status of COVID-19 related plastics and their potential impact on human health. *Current Opinion on Toxicology*, *27*, 47–53. https://doi.org/10.1016/j.cotox.2021.08.002

Goodman, K. E., Hare, J. T., Khamis, Z. I., Hua, T., & Sang, Q. X. A. (2021). Exposure of human lung cells to polystyrene microplastics significantly retards cell proliferation and triggers morphological changes. *Chemical Research in Toxicology*, *34*, 1069–1081.

Hiemstra, A., Rambonnet, L., Gravendeel, B., & Schilthuizen, M. (2021). The effects of COVID-19 litter on animal life. *Animal Biology*, 1–17. https://doi.org/10.1163/15707563-bja10052

Klemeš, J. J., Fan, Y. V., & Jiang, P. (2020). The energy and environmental footprints of COVID-19 fighting measures—PPE, disinfection, supply chains. *Energy*, *211*, 118701. https://doi.org/10.1016/j.energy.2020.118701

Kögel, T., Bjorøy, Ø., Toto, B., Bienfait, A. M., & Sanden, M. (2020). Micro- and nanoplastic toxicity on aquatic life: Determining factors. *Science of the Total Environment*, *709*, 136050. https://doi.org/10.1016/j.scitotenv.2019.136050

Kumar, H., Azad, A., Gupta, A., Sharma, J., Bherwani, H., Labhsetwar, N. K., & Kumar, R. (2020). COVID-19 Creating another problem? Sustainable solution for PPE disposal through LCA approach. *Environment, Development and Sustainability*, *23*(6), 9418–9432. https://doi.org/10.1007/s10668-020-01033-0

Lavers, J. L., Sharp, P. B., Stuckenbrock, S., & Bond, A. L. (2020). Entrapment in plastic debris endangers hermit crabs. *Journal of Hazardous Materials*, *387*, 121703. https://doi.org/10.1016/j.jhazmat.2019.121703

Muthuraman, Y., & Lakshminarayanan, I. (2021). A review of the COVID-19 pandemic and its interaction with environmental media. *Environmental Challenges*, *3*, 100040. https://doi.org/10.1016/j.envc.2021.100040

Neto, H. G., Bantel, C. G., Browning, J., Fina, N. D., Ballabio, T. A., Santana, F. T., de Karam E Britto, M., & Barbosa, C. B. (2021). Mortality of a juvenile Magellanic penguin (*Spheniscus magellanicus*, Spheniscidae) associated with the ingestion of a PFF-2 protective mask during the Covid-19 pandemic. *Marine Pollution Bulletin*, *166*, 112232. https://doi.org/10.1016/j.marpolbul.2021.112232

Prata, J. C., da Costa, J. P., Lopes, I., Duarte, A. C., & Rocha-Santos, T. (2020). Environmental exposure to microplastics: An overview on possible human health effects. *Science of the Total Environment*, *702*, 134455. https://doi.org/10.1016/j.scitotenv.2019.134455

Rahman, M. M., Bodrud-Doza, M., Griffiths, M. D., & Mamun, M. A. (2020). Biomedical waste amid COVID-19: Perspectives from Bangladesh. *The Lancet Global Health*, *8*(10), e1262. https://doi.org/10.1016/s2214-109x(20)30349-1

Samanta, P., Dey, S., & Ghosh, A. R. (2021). Are population size and diverse climatic conditions the driving factors for next COVID-19 pandemic epicenter in India? *Results in Physics*, *26*, 104454. https://doi.org/10.1016/j.rinp.2021.104454

Samanta, P., & Ghosh, A. R. (2021). Environmental perspectives of COVID-19 outbreaks—A review. *World Journal of Gastroenterology*, *27*(35), 5822–5850. https://doi.org/10.3748/wjg.v27.i35.5822

Shammi, M., & Tareq, S. M. (2021). Environmental catastrophe of COVID-19: Disposal and management of PPE in Bangladesh. *Global Social Welfare*, *8*(2), 133–136.

Shi, Q., Tang, J., Wang, L., Liu, R., & Giesy, J. P. (2021). Combined cytotoxicity of polystyrene nanoplastics and phthalate esters on human lung epithelial A549 cells and its mechanism. *Ecotoxicology and Environmental Safety*, *213*, 112041. https://doi.org/10.1016/j.ecoenv.2021.112041

Torres, F. G., Dioses-Salinas, D. C., Pizarro-Ortega, C. I., & De-la-Torre, G. E. (2021). Sorption of chemical contaminants on degradable and non-degradable microplastics: Recent progress and research trends. *Science of the Total Environment*, *757*, 143875. https://doi.org/10.1016/j.scitotenv.2020.143875

Tripathi, A., Tyagi, V. K., Vivekanand, V., Bose, P., & Suthar, S. (2020). Challenges, opportunities and progress in solid waste management during COVID-19 pandemic. *Case Studies in Chemical and Environmental Engineering*, *2*, 100060. https://doi.org/10.1016/j.cscee.2020.100060

Wang, X. W., Li, J. S., Zhen, B., Kong, Q. X., Song, N., & Xiao, W. J. (2005). Study on the resistance of severe acute respiratory syndrome-associated coronavirus. *Journal of Virological Methods*, *126*, 171–177.

Index

For Product Safety Concerns and Information please contact our EU representative GPSR@taylorandfrancis.com Taylor & Francis Verlag GmbH, Kaufingerstraße 24, 80331 München, Germany

Batch number: 10425309

Printed by Printforce, the Netherlands